RACISM AND ANTI-SEMITISM IN THE MENTAL HEALTH SYSTEM

By the survivors themselves

FOREWORD BY
FARZANA KHAN

COMPLIED BY DOLLY SEN

EDITED BY DR CASSANDRA LOVELOCK
& DEBRA SHULKES

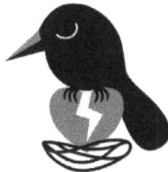

First published 2024

British Library Cataloguing in Publication data: a
catalogue record for this book is available from the
British Library.

© Dr Cassandra Lovelock, Debra Shulkes and Dolly Sen
COVER DESIGN: Caroline Cardus

ISBN 978-1-7393589-6-9
Ebook ISBN 978-1-7393589-5-2

WWW.CUCKOONESTBOOKS.CO.UK

Funded by

UNLIMITED **wellcome
collection**

Dedicated to the memory of the most wonderful, beautiful, kind and glorious Debra Shulkes (1975-2022)

CONTENTS

FOREWORD BY FARZANA KHAN

INTRODUCTION BY DR CASSANDRA LOVELOCK

STORIES OF RACISM AND DEHUMANISATION

STORIES OF RACISM IN MENTAL HEALTH SERVICES

STORIES OF BEING IN RACIALISED BODY

CONTRIBUTORS

BIRDSONG TEAM

THANKS AND ACKNOWLEDGMENTS

GLOSSARY

INDEX

OUR GROUP MESSAGE TO ANYONE HOLDING ELITIST OPINIONS (written by Cassandra Lovelock)

"Peoples' stories are their own, in whatever form they have been put across in this book. For that reason, I beg you to take your elitist opinions and shove them up your ass. These books are not grammatically perfect, it has not softened itself for our readers, and we have not asked our authors to reshape themselves to fit into already formed constructs and narratives about mental health. This is not an academic book, though every academic should read it and weep."

FOREWORD by Farzana Khan

The only way to begin and travel through this book is to invite ourselves to the intentional act of listening.

Take a moment here to prepare to listen.

Prepare your space, prepare your focus, prepare your body, prepare at the top of each page.

When I was invited to write the foreword of this book, the task felt profound and important, I was being entrusted with testimonies of deeply personal and powerful acts of courage and truth-telling. Stories that are powerful, painful, traumatic, defiant, heart-breaking, brave, tender, strong, fierce, and bold. They demand us to listen and many times throughout this book, we come across the plea and protest of the very human and fundamental need of wanting to be heard. From the 'battle to be heard' to the number of times, these testimonies evidence being 'dismissed', 'unheard', 'ignored', being made to feel people's pain and experiences are 'unspeakable' and that 'no one listened'. Therefore, it matters that we attend to this book as a practice of deeper listening and witnessing to the multitudes of experiences especially voiced by those through racism we are trained to ignore or diminish.

We live in a world organised to consume, scroll, pass by, readying to speak back, react, critique without offering each other the witnessing and humanising that deep listening gives us. In the UK and British society, it's deemed 'British' to have a 'stiff upper lip' or to avoid complex and emotive spaces and our institutions, including public health, reinforce this too.

We are less practised to hold, to hear, to sit with, to dwell on. These are not just cultural tropes but extend to and emerge from a colonial, patriarchal and capitalist logic that relies on compartmentalising us, regulating our emotional and connective capacities as inferior and signs of 'barbarity', 'hysterics' or the 'uncivilised', which then consolidates into racist, classist, ableist etc mechanics amongst us and our public institutions. We become socialised to not hear and value each other and to do this even less for those racialised, people who are made structurally and systemically unheard, erased and invisibilised. In a similar vein our society is designed in a deeply ableist way that sick, disabled and distressed people also experience erasure and being ignored. The consequences of this is how much our society, public infrastructures, public bodies including health systems are set up to fail Black and people of colour and disabled, sick and distressed people because of this habitual unhearing and unseeing that keeps us unknown and un-met. Breaking these intimate and structural cycles of failing people, especially when they are most in need, means we find new ways of listening. Alongside this we have to be interrogating which voices are valued? What informs our ideas of who is worth listening to and not? What knowledge is important and considered valid? Who benefits and who is harmed from these ideas?

This book was an intentional act of forefronting and affirming the voices of those with living experiences of racism and experiences of mental distress as valid. As acts of expanding what we think we know, as ways of showing up the gaps in our thinking and as ways of bridging some of those unknowns.

These insights enrich not only the types of care people get but support us to really attend to one another in the most appropriate and humanised way. Without this we continue, as seen throughout this book, the structural and personal entrapments that are the experiences of Black and People of colour within mental health settings and further from school to housing, to policing and beyond. If we listen carefully, we can arrange our societies and health provisions differently and more robustly. As informed by the first Healing Justice Principle;

'We begin by listening"[1]

Take a moment, a breath and beat at any moment you need to.

FARZANA KHAN, Writer and Social Sculptor

---

[1] https://justhealing.files.wordpress.com/2012/04/hjps-guidingprinciples.pdf

—

INTRODUCTION - Dr Cassandra Lovelock

This book forms part of an Unlimited and Wellcome Collection funded project which aims to explore the current archived narratives on mental health. Dolly says she hopes it does some way to ease the trauma of mental health system survivors – having their truth held up to the same level as the clinical narratives which see us as a problem with a solution rather than a person.

Asking people to recount their experiences of racism can be harrowing, retraumatising, and just incredibly sad. Peoples' stories are their own, in whatever form they have been put across in this book. For that reason, I beg you to take your elitist opinions and shove them up your ass. This book is not grammatically perfect, it has not softened itself for our readers, and we have not asked our authors to reshape themselves to fit into already formed constructs and narratives about mental health. This is not an academic book, though every academic should read it and weep.

On the same note, we are not going to police our authors for the language choices they have made when referring to their communities. We could write another book on whether BAME or BME or racialised communities or global majority is the correct term, but the space we have tried to make in these books is one of healing, grounding, and restoration of people's truths. Truths which the system often strips away.

It was not until recently that NHS mental health services acknowledged that experiencing racism is a form of trauma. Just as recently, with the murder of George Floyd, the world seemed to remember that existing in a racist society is something inherently traumatic; white people were reminded racism was not fixed in 1960s and fled to the comfort of performative activism.

—

With black squares littering Instagram and twitter as white people decided to 'blackout' to show their support for Black lives I am left wonder what do black squares do for Black lives?

The voices of those living in racialised bodies are lost within mental health narratives. Drowned out by more easily digestible stories which do not force the uncomfortable but merely push at the edges of comfort. We have become numb to the statistics that categorise our lives. We can recite them, have watched politicians recite them for personal gain, and mental health services do it every time they claim lessons are 'learned'.

Black people are 5 times more likely than white peoples to be detained under the mental health act; with 344 detentions per 100,000 of people compared to just 75 per 100,000 with Black African people had the highest rate of detention among ethnic groups[2]

Everyone one of those detentions was a racialised person having their rights stripped away. Judge on scales that we did not know existed never mind we were being judged upon until we failed. Each detention is a person's story, a person with a name, a life and at least one person they share it with. But the thing that connects them all together was the fact they were racialised, that the colour of their skin, the structure of their features entitled them to the most barbaric treatment our mental health system has.

- Racialised people are most likely to be placed under section 136 with Black or Black British people experiencing section 136 69 uses per 100,000 people.

---

[2] (UK Gov, 2022: Detentions under the Mental Health Act)

—

- Racialised people are more likely to be victims of coercive practices, uses of force and violence, and restraint practices. [3]

'Seni's Law' (otherwise known as the Mental Health units Use of Force Act 2018) is the shoulders that all racialised people stand upon in our fight for treatment over violence. Olaseni Lewis known as Seni is the name we chant and the scream and use when looking and mourning for the lost lives of racialised people due to and within the mental health system. Seni's life is one of many racialised and particular Black men's lives lost to acts of violence in the mental health system. Say his name. Scream it for every person who is restrained. We are restrained and we are killed. Murdered by the people we beg for help when we have nowhere else to turn. There are stories within every statistic you just have to listen.

We don't need statistics, though, to illustrate why psychiatry – and within that UK mental health services are a weapon for the maintenance of white supremacy. Psychiatry has a long history starting with 'biological psychiatry' or racial hygiene and eugenics. Psychiatrists played a crucial role in Eugenics – particularly within Nazi Germany and the United States.

---

[3] (NHS Digital, 2022 Mental Health Act Statistics 2021-22)

Hitler signed a document called *'The Law for the Prevention of Offspring with Hereditary Diseases.'* This law was designed to prevent the continuation of 'mental retardation,' schizophrenia, and alcoholism in the Aryan German population via forced sterilisation, children with deformities being killed and "Action T4" – a euthanasia program that entailed the targeted killing of adult psychiatric patients via gas, lethal injections, or starvation[4].

The American eugenics movement was firmly rooted in the biological determinist ideas of Francis Galton who believed in selective breeding of the human species. He and his followers advocated for involuntary sterilization and restrictive laws for marriage and immigration focusing on the mentally ill and those from racialised communities to ensure the purity of Americans.

In 1927, the U.S. Supreme Court enabled states to determine who was allowed to have children, in essence allow eugenics to be enforced by state laws. These family laws prohibited the marriage of "lunatics," "imbeciles," "epileptics," the "insane," and the "weak minded" as well as having significant cross over with what Black and other racialised people's rights to have children. Some of these laws lingered in different states of the union in one way or another until 1980s[5],[6].

---

[4] Udo B. Euthanasia in Germany Before and During the Third Reich. Heric AB, Radosh L. trans. Münster: Klemm und Oelschläger; (2010). Chapter 4, p. 597–9)

[5] (Ian Robert D. *Keeping America Sane: Psychiatry and Eugenics in the United States Canada, 1880-1940.* New York: Cornell University Press; (1997).

[6] Samuel Jan B, Parry J, Weiner BA. *The Mentally Disabled and the Law.* 3rd ed Chicago: American Bar Foundation; (1985). p. 10–1

Arriving at the system we have now, then, one built off the cis-het non-disabled white man being the ideal. One which, particularly in the USA, Britain, and Germany never even attempted to divorced itself from these eugenicist principles. A system that forced sterilisation and murder of racialised people with mental illness. Psychiatry has always been a weapon for those in power to use to uphold white supremacy and the voices in this book are the ones living everyday paying that price. Psychiatry has caused and continues to cause great pain to generations of people, and there are not many places they can say this without being punished for it, or not taken seriously, or believed.

Why won't the Mental Health System face its racism?

Psychiatry and every player within the mental health system – I mean the police, I mean social workers, I mean policy makers and researchers, mental health practitioners and clinicians, civil servants, every last one of them... and myself I suppose as one of them; we have an ongoing, long term developmental disregard for the lives of Black, brown and those living in racialised bodies. It started with eugenicist principles granting the system permission to decide who is worthy. It is pervasive and ongoing now; we still decide who is worthy.

How someone enters the mental health system brands whether you are a good or bad service user. It is a pervasive factor in how you will experience it, and how for racialised groups who frequently enter the mental health system as a 'problem' this is devastating. We are pushed into the system as a problem, a stain, as something outside of medical textbooks. We are branded criminals or we are asylum seekers, or we have arrived at the door step of the mental health system through safe-guarding. We are problem to be fixed not a person to be support.

The 'model minority' permeates psychiatric care to varying degrees. White supremacy has positioned certain racialised minorities as better than the others. Whether that better is blending into white society, traditional achievements such as academics, or the best at not 'burdening' the system the 'Model Minorities' that whiteness shoves toward racialised people as aspirational is dangerous it infiltrates our thinking too. We must perform whiteness to be seen as human, we must try on our whiteness and forget who and where we are for even an ounce of compassion. We must act like that one random racialised person this psychiatrist is comparing us too in the hopes of even a percentage of treatment – We've all heard it before

'I've treated a bunch of mixed people before and they responded well. So why aren't you?'

Like we are some monoliths. Racialised or white. That's all the system can see.

How do we make race in mental health more than a talking point?

Why is the answer to this question getting people to 'whore out' their trauma? Why does it take a Black person after brown person after East Asian person after Jewish person on cycle to expose the most intimate and vulnerable parts of ourselves to people who say that they care. Exposing our truths to the people that hold the power to make a difference in any of our lives. Why do we have to remind them that we are human? Why are they so able to negate our realities and humanity if it doesn't fit with the narrative they have? Every day they walk on a history littered with Black and brown bodies while 'committing' to be an anti-racist.

I resent the idea that my skin colour grants people permission to treat me as less than. I resent the idea that the features which mark my skin somehow allow those with more power to squash me and mould me into whatever they please. I resent the idea that my resistance to this is either seen as inspirational or a reason to pathologise me.

I consider every psychiatric label I receive a celebration of my subversion from the Whiteness I am expected to assimilate into. Every psychiatric label I am given re-affirms my breaking away and unlearning of the whiteness I desperately clawed for in a culture which declared I was not worthy.

I cannot end this intro and I have not edited these books without acknowledging the fact that I am standing on the shoulders of giants. The people who took on the mental health system head on. Don't just say their names scream them.

This book makes space for the stories which exist in between the statistics. The stories which form the talking points that white people use to judge our lives. For the kids who looked in the mirror and begged to be different, to be white. This book shares the pain and anguish of being seen as less than human. It is place for the beauty of Black excellent, of Brown Joy, of Jewish brilliance, and the merits of every person who lives in a racialised body to flourish.

Be proud of yourselves. We will endure. We will flourish.

STORIES OF RACISM
AND DEHUMANISATION

PSYCHIATRY DOESN'T LOVE BLACK OR BROWN PEOPLE – Dolly Sen

It was a spring morning, approaching Easter. The sun was out, and the air bright but cool. I was about 4 years old. We had just moved into a new house but we weren't allowed to go into the garden because of the previous cold weather. My mum went out there to set up a washing line and took me and my sister with her. My sister and I slid down the washing line pole as if we were firefighters, making siren noises as we ran around. Suddenly I felt something wet on me. I looked up to see a man with a moustache, who lived next door, leaning over the fence: "Shut up, you dirty brown mongrels!" And he spat on me again. This was my first memory of racism, although I didn't really understand it as such at the time. I just thought I was thing to be disgusted by, and as I was already getting that message from my abusive father, I took it on as truth.

Move forward a year or two, I am at school. Most of the other kids are ok. One or two call me 'Paki' and tell me to go back to where I come from. No teacher tells them off. This thing called racism is a hard thing to understand as a child, but what you do understand is that you are the other, the alien; there is something about you that people hate when all you wanted to do was play with some toys.

Aged about 10, I am visiting Brick Lane in the East End with my dad. He and the friend he's visiting sit down for a drink. His friend ushers his kids out the house and tells them to take me with them.

His son and daughter show me around their neighbourhood and as we turn a corner, we are confronted by a gang of white children and teenagers. The daughter drags me by the arm and shouts "Run!" I do what she says as the gang of white kids begins to chase after us, threatening to "kick our paki heads in". We manage to jump into a tower block lift and watch the doors slide dramatically closed as our pursuers get within a few inches of the lift. Why do they hate us? What did I do? What is wrong with me?

One night in 1981 the whole family is travelling on an old route master bus. We're coming back to Streatham from an Easter party organised by social services for Deaf people and their families. The bus does not take its usual route, instead taking a displaced one avoiding Brixton. My dad asks the conductor what's going on. "There's some trouble in Brixton." Once home, we put the news on. There are images of Brixton burning; I recognise parts I've walked through with my mum when we go shopping. People on TV are talking about criminal elements and the poor moral attitudes of the rioters. But living near Brixton I've also heard the other side, of people fed up with police harassment, fed up with being badly treated by authorities, of being spat at because of their colour.

My dad was racist himself. He called the rioting looters "black thieving bastards" even though he will go down to the Brixton shops the next day to see if there's anything else worth nicking.

All this is confusing for a child. My dad has made me scared of Black people. But from our third-floor flat, overlooking the main road, I have also seen the police stop Black people for no reason, and use physical violence on younger Black men who were not physically threatening, just vocal in their anger.

Who was right or wrong about the world? Who were the good guys? Police, school, adults, my parents were meant to be, but they scared me, and none of them could offer safety to the very scared child that was me.

Coupled with this is the fact that I am of mixed heritage: my dad Indian and my mum Scots-Irish. I never felt I belonged anywhere. There was also some unknown war waging itself inside me. I have oppressor and oppressed DNA in me. My white great-great-grandfather served in the British Army in India, where my Indian ancestors were being brutalised and treated like second-class citizens. Which part of my mind do I de-colonise first? How do I do that anyway? Who can teach me to do that?

I did not have only one form of trauma whilst growing up. My abusive father taught me that I was worthless, that there was something wrong with me. This bled into the auditory hallucinations I experienced from the age of 14; with the content of my voices being derogatory and brutal; telling me I should kill myself because I shouldn't be around, that nobody liked me. The voices echoed my abusers' words: whenever I experienced racism, I had that same sense of being unaccepted, hated, demonised and defective, all this giving fuel to the voices.

Racism is part of the 'shitty committee' that holds conversations in my head and breaks my heart, continually. Not only that, it fed the thinking that I was an alien from out of space which led me to being hospitalised for the first time on a psychiatric ward. On the hospital ward, it was Black people who were controlled and restrained more than everyone else. It seemed like they were being punished purely for the colour of their skin, which to me was insanity. How crazy-making it is when the institution that professes to be the figurehead of sanity is acting in such a delusional and unsound way.

Racism in the mental health system has been there since its beginning. Psychiatry has grown out of a soil that is nourished with white supremacy and colonialism. It doesn't want to acknowledge that. Psychiatry has no insight into its own condition. It is a danger to itself and others.

The mental health system is an ugly machine that takes in Black and Brown people and is happy and willing to send them out in coffins through control and restraint, or drive them into those coffins through encouraging self-hatred.

One of the things I want to put across with these three Birdsong books is that we must stop insisting mental distress is an illness that originates in the brain, for many of us it is an injury or wound. The mental health system has to accept this, and step one is to identify the weapons that keep wounding people. But psychiatry won't admit that one of the armaments is the system itself. It can't afford to admit to mental distress as a wound. Racism is a trauma, a laceration, an abrasion on the softest part of the human being, it is a heartbreaker. It is a wrongdoing, an affront, a grievance. It loves to jettison responsibility by individualising the mental distress, blaming it on the people who have been hurt rather than the outside forces that injured them. The racist mental health system adds to your pain, and then pathologises you for that pain, all the while insisting it is not racist. My saving grace was learning to return that hatred to sender. Self-disgust is one of the weapons 'gifted' to people by brutal persons and regimes to keep us in our place.

I learnt over the years to dispense with self-hatred. I am now left with the rage that fuels my creativity and activism. Now my creativity and activism has brought me to this book.

That is not to say racism still doesn't cause me pain. The current war in Ukraine is heart-breaking and this country opening its arms to let in its refugees is a beautiful thing. But by the same token, Britain is happy to watch Brown and Black people drown in the channel. This double standard may be hard to inhabit if you are white. Just imagine what it is like if you are Brown or Black and British? How can you trust any white stranger? What if they would prefer you dead? How can the mental health system disregard all this as unimportant and then expect you to trust it? How do I know the system treats racism as immaterial? In the many decades of my being in the system, not one clinician has asked how racism has impacted my mental health, or how many times it has broken my already bruised heart. It is a bit like seeing a person on fire, saying nothing about the flames, and asking them to be more resilient *or to do some mindfulness.* The system needs to do some minefield-ness first: to stop planting deadly traps and make safe the terrain of people's identity and sense of self.

You will not find a single mention of the system's own bigotry in my patient notes but you will see its own racism. In just the last few years, I have had many ethnicities recorded because nobody has bothered to ask me. You will see demeaning language used to deny the pain of whenever I have been the brunt of prejudice and discrimination. In those recent notes, you will read that 'Dolly has claimed she has experienced racism', and other such dismissive phrases.

As long as psychiatry wants to make people ugly, the pain will continue and the truth of our lives will be left behind. Our patient notes do not tell our stories. They are merely a screenshot of which ever racist practitioner decided it was worth noting down that day. How many Black and Brown people are labelled as monsters in the system? How many have their lives ruined by the very structure that is meant to save them? How come I can see the magnificence and spirit of racialised people trying to reclaim their stories, lives, and dignity, but services can't? The mental health system does not lean in to try and hear the faint birdsong there. They should; it is beautiful.

We have to be the singer and the song for those who have forgotten how to sing and those who have been silenced forever. Let the quiet birds sing. One day we will drown out the hunters. We have to. I am tired of seeing the pile of bodies of the dead.

I'VE BEEN EVERYWHERE BUT NEVER GOT ANYWHERE – Questions for Conne Artist

What caused your distress?

I was born in Paris in the mid-seventies in a Tunisian family. We lived in overcrowded conditions. From as early as I can remember I was worried about money and day to day survival. My biggest obsessions were survival, finding money, and saving my family from overcrowding, poverty and mental illness.

I felt very responsible for my family and, as the last one who arrived on the scene, I had a sense that I needed to adapt to the way things were at home, taking what I was given and not asking too many questions.

We lived in an old building and didn't have a toilet or bathroom inside our small one-bedroom flat. Instead we had to share an outside bathroom with our next-door neighbours, a couple of retired French people. Being the youngest, I was always very eager to catch up with my siblings and be able to do as much as they could. In the cold and dark outside toilet to which I ran to relieve myself, I deciphered some of the first words I ever read on hanging handwritten signs. As well as reading 'please clean after yourself', there were smaller scribbles and signs which read 'Arabs stink' or 'go home'.

These racist messages were some of the first things I have ever read and became etched onto my consciousness, an underlying anxiety and frantic despair that would be present all my life. I was not wanted here. I needed to find somewhere I could be allowed to live.

Within my family, I felt equally alienated as I was often reminded that I needed to take as little space as possible. Though I am sure that everyone had love for me, I was very conscious that my arrival had made the family's cramped conditions worse and that I needed to somehow make myself scarce. My mother, also believing that she was keeping me safe, told me that Arabs were not welcome in France and that, if I was to ever have a toy that a French white kid wanted, I needed to let them have it, as it was 'their country and not ours.'

On television too, I heard the same message from Jean Marie Le Pen, the national front leader whose presidential campaign motto had been: 'France: love it or leave it'. He was foaming at the mouth, was extremely hateful of North African migrants like my family, and was constantly comparing us to dangerous vermin or a cancer that was 'eating' France.

I must have been about 4 when I heard this frightening rhetoric from the white hateful man with the eye patch and I remember deciding that I would leave France just as soon as I could. I felt unwanted everywhere I went and proceeded to make myself scarce by being a straight A student and acting as the mascot in my family, making it my duty to work daily at making sure everyone was okay and reconciling warring parties all around me. People, like rats in a bucket, will not get on very well when space is scarce, so we all developed coping strategies to bear with the situation. Mine was to escape through books and fantasy. By focusing on others, I stopped paying attention to what I was feeling, prompting a lifelong dissociative state, where I have no idea of what I am feeling and my body is in the room but I am not. This is frequent, I hear, for people living with complex PTSD. I never felt normal and have spent a lifetime feeling there was so much that was wrong with me.

School was tough. My nappy hair was mocked by disgusted children and it was assumed that brown people like myself were dirty. I felt unable to cleanse myself of 'my dirt', which, as often implied through the hostile environment, was deeply ingrained in me, as I was an Arab.

Throughout these very difficult years, we kept hoping for a better future through our yearly visits to Tunisia where my parents were building a house. Life in France was very difficult and our holidays in Tunisia were full of sunshine, space and family love.

Every year I kept asking my mum when we were going back and it was always 'next year' but around age 12, I finally understood that we were not going back and that life in France was all there really was. I became overwhelmed by an obsession with suicide, which I saw as the only possible way out to such a painful existence. Slowly, I did less well at school, became more introverted and started looking for ways to self-harm, cutting myself. I also started hanging out with older kids and discovered alcohol. I felt awful every day, crying and wanting to hide. I started avoiding school and went to hang out with a bunch of older kids who hung out with local punks. We drank cheap beer from the same bottle. I liked how the alcohol and drugs seemed to make the pain recede. I was comfortably numb and nothing mattered anymore.

I continued on this path, caught between the strict expectations of my Tunisian parents and the impossibility of ever finding my place in France, as long as I looked as I did, had my Arab sounding name, and nothing to look forward to. I was taken to the mental hospital when I was 15 and then another a year later. That's where I first got acquainted with psychiatric pills, which I started to use alongside alcohol to regulate my emotions and sometimes press 'stop'. I would hate waking up after yet another failed suicide attempt. Though I never thought I would end up in a mental hospital when I was younger, I discovered that there was a place ready for a brown girl like me all along. I understood that it had been expected that I would not amount to anything as the daughter of Arab migrants, and the hospital seemed like a place where I could live away from home for years. I met many people who looked like myself and who had settled for that. Psychiatric treatment in France was still very old fashioned and it seemed normal to lock a kid in with grown adults who had been in the system for years, so I saw quite a few things I shouldn't have.

I finally managed to escape the mental hospital shortly before I turned 18, but by this time I needed pills and alcohol to just about feel ok. I still took overdoses at times to turn the lights out for several days and silence my anguish.

I moved further away from interacting with my family, living with boyfriends, hanging out in squats, and punk gigs. When my dad died, I spiralled out of control and my mental health got much worse. I met the father of my kids and moved to London.

Your experience in the British mental health system - how did it make you feel?

The Mental Health system made me feel dirty and ashamed for feeling the way I did. As an isolated disabled migrant non-white single mother, I always felt the thinly veiled threats that if I wasn't coping, my children would then be taken away. How is that for an incentive to feel better…. immediately?

It is that pressure that has made me feel more unwell than what I would have probably been, all this hiding, all this masquerading. Because of my intersectionality, I was doomed, and my children were looked at as unfortunates, at school and at play. There were frequent incursions by concerned social services, coming in to check that the children were not 'at risk'. I have constantly reached out for help throughout my children's childhood but never received the support I needed. Instead, I was offered additional servings of stigma through the criminalising lens of 'we need to check that you're coping' for the children's sake. I sought to self-medicate my enormous pain through using drugs and alcohol and also self-harming at home when the kids were in bed.

When I sought help for my addictions through 12 step programs, I was again scrutinised and told that the authorities needed to check if the children were okay. As far as I knew, the children were okay but I wasn't. I was not offered any help whatsoever and me being isolated without friends or family, made me feel like a target for the authorities to continually investigate.

As I felt so vulnerable and alone, in a hostile environment with my two daughters, I always looked impeccable, with my bright red lipstick, perfume and smart clothes. *'Looking good'* was the number one trick I had picked up from growing up not being wanted in France, where I learnt to have less going against me by presenting an impeccable image.

In the context of the mental health system, I was never believed for the distress I described mainly because the bar in accessing help was so high that I did not qualify for getting any support. I could read in many a bemused psychiatrist's eye the disbelief at having a client looking like myself supposedly being on the brink of yet another crisis. I could tell that my pain was not taken seriously as I was not foaming at the mouth or soiling myself. I was eventually sent on my way with a Borderline Personality Disorder (BPD) diagnosis, a dustbin label that gets handed to thousands of people, pushing them into a lifetime of hardship, from being denied benefits to being offered no help.

With that 'magic label', I ended up even more stranded and stigmatised, as now, I would only be able to access the Highgate mental health centre which was specialising in treating those who got given that label. Highgate mental health centre was a horrible and cold place where BPD patients attended as outpatients. The 'care' consisted of mentalisation and mindfulness sessions mainly teaching you to cope with the heightened anxiety and emotions which are a side effect of having experienced multiple traumas. There were also group therapy sessions where some of us were deemed to be doing very well, whilst others, like myself, weren't. The therapist in charge of these groups captained a highly dysfunctional ship and would let some people get away with all sorts of stuff, whilst others, like myself, were not welcome to speak.

The 'care' was so bad there that a girl who was a bit larger and possibly suffering from an eating disorder was told by the therapist at the group sessions that 'she took too much space'. This girl later killed herself, possibly because of the cold clinical 'care' offered at Highgate mental health centre. Suicide is sadly a common occurrence in the MH system and they seem to have quotas for how many collaterals jump off the endless cycle of state-sanctioned abuse every year. I owe my life to having stopped attending these groups and not engaging in that type of 'care'.

I carried on asking for help for decades through my GP, who sent me to the psychiatrist who would send me to therapists who would send me back to the GP. A few years ago, I stopped asking for help as I finally accepted that there was none available. I have been parked on the same medication for the past two decades and though it has not worked for some time, I have ended up in A&E every time I tried to stop.

Did you find the Mental Health System racist? If so, how so?

At Highgate mental health centre's group session, a young, blonde, white woman took over the sessions, looking at the floor and saying that she felt intimidated by me. She had previously said that she felt anxious that she may lose her job because of her mental health. I had responded that at least she had a job and that she was probably doing better than she realised. To my horror, she had heard me saying that 'I hated her for having a job and that her job should have been mine', something along those lines.

Unbelievably, when I protested and said that I had never said such a thing, the therapist agreed that this was what I had said. The whole group followed suit. I was infuriated and I could see that I stepped right into a role that had been there all along for me: 'the angry brown female'. I forced myself to attend a couple more sessions, believing that some 'shitty Highgate mental health centre care' was better than no 'care' at all but my saving grace was to leave the group.

I had been self-harming since that and when I returned there, was forced to sit in silence, being blanked or glared at by the group whilst the fragile young white woman stared at the floor, shook in her boots and complained with a barely-there voice to the group about being scared because I was in the room. Being cast as a bully and a villain was definitely motivated by the fact that I was not white and it chimed with the whole experiences I had had growing up in France where I was deemed wrong no matter what I did or didn't do.

I felt crushed when I fully realised the extent of systemic oppression. When I reached my forties and up at the onset of yet another crisis, I saw how schools, doctors, social services, and the police worked hand in hand to label and exclude my family, painting us as dysfunctional.

We were poor, non-white and isolated, so here again, we got offered more labels, less love and more judgment.

When I broke down in tears at my daughter's primary school's headteacher's office, I instantly knew I had committed a grave mistake. He was a progressive Black gay headteacher, so I thought I may get some empathy from him but when I let him know how much I was struggling, I immediately sensed the room close down on me.

From then on, my family got ostracised, my kids got scrutinised as problem kids who could potentially be 'at risk'. No help was given but judgement and ostracisation became the norm. I was looked at as a concern and my kids were blamed and shamed for all sorts of things other kids wouldn't get in trouble for.

2014 was a clusterfuck. It was the culmination of years of struggling on my own, bleeding knuckles from knocking on doors, and asking for help. Both my daughters were bullied and so was I at work. The oversubscribed local secondary school had a field day with my family, casting us as the problem family whilst white British families of the bullies were left off the hook. My daughter was repeatedly physically attacked on her way to school, which gave me panic attacks.

Self-harm returned and I was a hot mess. Meanwhile, my eldest daughter was becoming very aggressive, and I struggled more and more with her. When I lost it one day and hit her, the doctor I sought help from referred me to the police, who urged me to accept a caution as a slap on the wrist instead of going to court.

The caution cost me the job I had secured to get out of the dysfunctional one I was trapped in. This job being withdrawn was the trigger for the obsession with suicide to return.

I felt like I had no way out and no way to rebuild my life. I had no rights to benefits, my eldest daughter was taken into state care, and I just wanted to die. We were cast as the stereotypical 'problematic family' and I was the 'aggressive brown woman'. No one ever spoke to us at any point to find out who we were. I was sent many social workers who would add into my stress by scrutinising my children, myself and our lifestyle and would then withdraw, without offering any support.

The agencies that should have supported me and my daughters came together to crush my family. I have no doubt whatsoever about systemic racism being at play here, as we were constantly perceived as deviant, cunning, and violent. No one had helped for decades and my exhaustion with the system became palpable. We have been on the receiving end of a brutal system designed to shame, punish, and exclude people like us, who don't fit in the boxes, people who were racialised, who had intersectional 'deviant' identities.

What would you have liked?

I would have liked being treated like an individual, being shown that I mattered, being shown that I was safe, instead of regarding my children as always potentially at risk because of my mental health. I would have liked to champion what I had instead of punished for what I lacked. It would have been nice, also, to be given support from the onset of feeling bad, not further down the line when a crisis is looming, and social services get involved.

In the future, I would like to be listened to, to be believed when I say I am hurting, to be treated as a human being, to be offered help when I say I need it, to be included, to be trusted when I report something. I would love it if people and authorities stopped assuming that I am always the one who is in the wrong. I would also appreciate not being picked on for my race and my disability. I would love to have my many talents and skills rewarded and get a secure livelihood. One day, I would love to be able to tell my story out loud without fear of repercussions but we're not there yet.

———

FOLLOWING IMAGES ARE BY CONNE

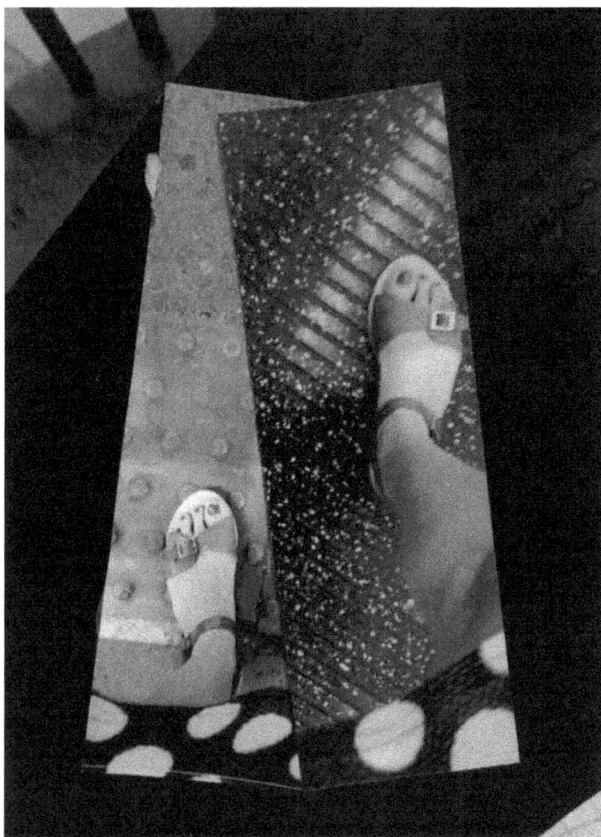

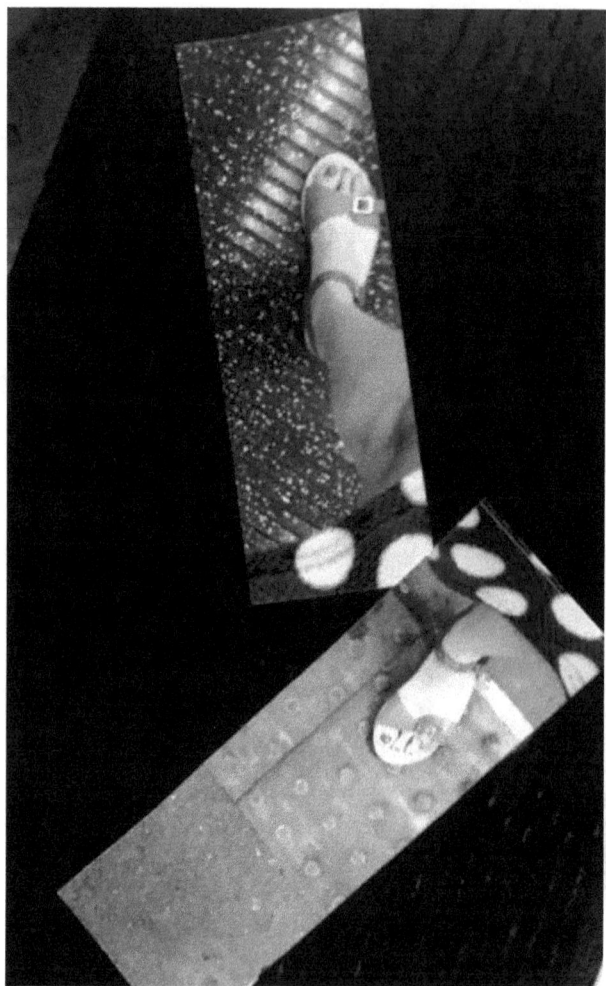

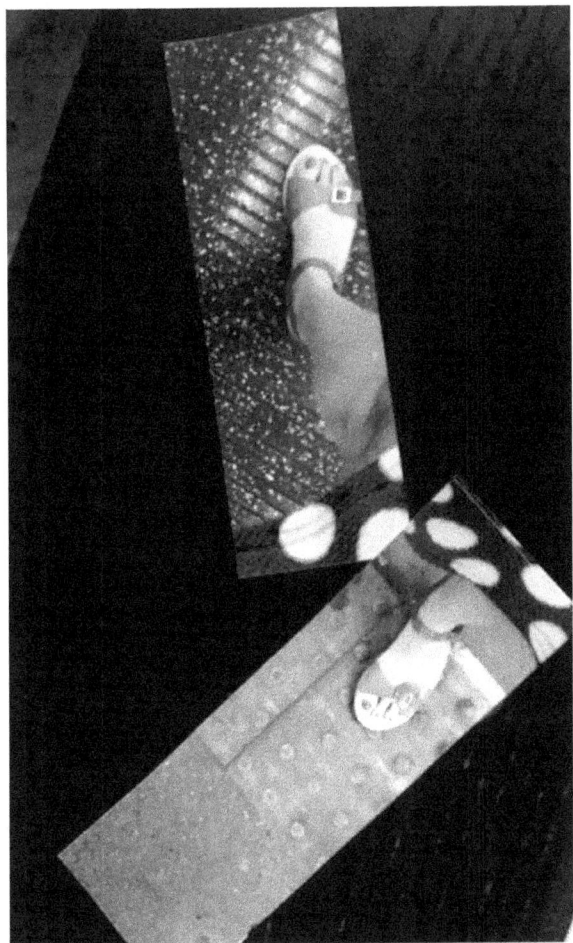

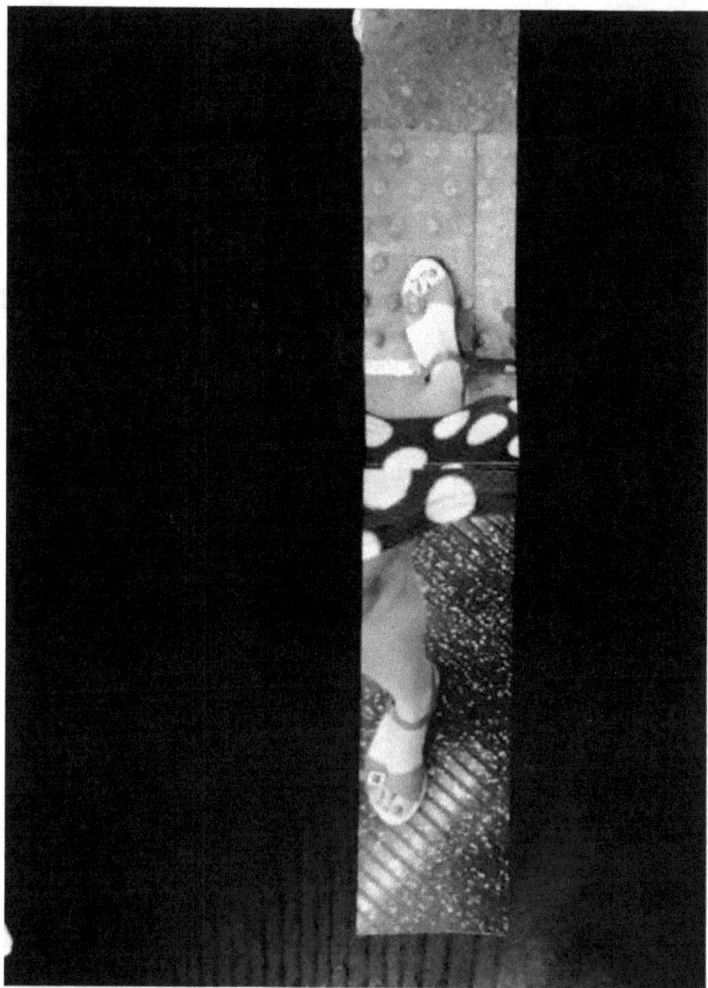

THERAPY – David Sohanpal

Coming to this country

I have been pondering on this issue for some time now, how is it that people do not speak out against unscrupulous practice from psychotherapists. It's time for me to speak out; as it has taken a toll on my life and drove me to trying to end my own life. After being diagnosed with PTSD, I went seeking help for my trauma but ended up more traumatised. Life has been a life roller-coaster and I'm even more damaged at the end.

I am an asylum seeker, a fugee, an immigrant, and brown man with no status. I come from a third world country which I had to flee as it illegal to speak out on oppression or stand up for human rights. As a result for standing up to these injustices I was brutally attacked, I received death threats. This has left me with panic attacks, depression, and PTSD which I buried deep inside me. Only when I got to the UK was it suggested I seek support from a therapist. I hoped they would help me deal with my depression and anxiety and panics but they did not.

I sought out support from a charity that supposedly specialises in supporting asylum seekers who have experienced trauma. But it was not the freedom from torture I thought it would be. It was a total nightmare, a living hell. They were a bunch of meretricious 'experts' and I am in worse off after I went to therapy with them. My mental health and confidence have deteriorated. Yes, I am new to all this therapy stuff in this country, I didn't know what to expect. I thought they would help me deal with the traumas I have been carrying all these years but they only amplified them.

I wasn't given or told of any written comprehension plan of how or what therapy that they would give. I just went along as I trusted them as they claimed to be the expert. This experience has put me off seeing any therapist in a while, it has made me more reclusive, it has scared me just thinking of it gives me nightmares. It has created these clouds of doubts of ever seeking help.

Therapists and being street homeless

In order for someone to become a therapist, I think they should have lived experience. They need to have been on the other side of the couch and not just learn through textbooks. The therapists at the charity definitely did not have sufficient or specific enough training to address my issues or treat my problems. Because my problems existed outside of the scope of 'normal' practice, they are not clearly defined, there is no easy way they can help me solve them whatever I bought to therapy. The therapist I had would shout at me to speak and tell me that her time is ticking. She acted so flipping insensitively, especially given she knew that I was street homeless.

There was a time I was attacked at night while I was sleeping in the park. By the time I had therapy I was still in shock, I didn't feel like talking. But the therapist kept pushing. She didn't understand what it's like to sleep outside below freezing, to have no access to public funds. It's like me, a man, telling a woman what it is like to give birth because I read about it in a book. How does that make me an expert when I have never and will never experience what it is like. The therapist was always pushing me to talk about things I was not ready to, she kept pushing a therapeutic approach rather than building trust first.

She was not sensitive to my needs nor could empathise that I was coming from a different culture. I was in a new country and was street homeless; that exclusion of feelings and somatic experience of which was amplifying my traumas.

The therapist didn't want to listen. She wasn't open to my knowledge of what was the cause and what is the solution for part of traumas. I needed people to give me the time, the space to grieve, to vent. Everyone is different and needs to come around at different times. This therapist didn't get it. I guess the books she learned through talk about just one person opening up within 2 sessions. But this doesn't mean everyone is ready to open up in the second session but when I wasn't she started shouting at me.

Beyond this she insisted on being overly friendly with me; trying to sit next to me when I was at social event and inappropriately touching me as if I need comforting. I felt gross and repulsed which even push me further not wanting to open up.

There was a time I collapsed in front of the charities building – they were so quick to jump to the conclusion that I had OD-ed. They could have simply read the discharge note I had which would have told them the reason I was there that night was because I had been harassed in the place I had bedded down for the night; I had walked in the cold, on an empty stomach and that is reason why I collapsed, I was tired, I was exhausted. The fact they couldn't be bothered to even look at this doctor's note which did take into account my street homelessness in my needs. This charity couldn't figure out that having a place to feel safe at night would help me. Instead I was stuck with a charity ran by meretricious racist people.

It's weird that these 'expert therapists' at this 'expert charity' did not understand that being street homeless was traumatic. That it will be harder for me to recover if I am stuck in this situation. As I was street homeless and was sleeping only a few hours each night, I was worried about experiencing mania but when I told my therapist she ignored it. When I asked for a tent so I could have somewhere safer to sleep without being moved on, they said no. The charity apparently said it would 'spoil their image.' They were more concerned about their image, the façade, than helping an actual human being. Any time I would make suggestions that would help my situation I was constantly belittled. Talking to me like I don't know what is best for me. The therapists kept telling me how and what I should feel but they only knew from reading books.

Therapists and state help

When I was given emergency accommodation by Home Office I was very apprehensive to go. Upon arrival I was shown to my room which had no windows and the carpet smelt like some had just urinated on it, the bed had bed bugs and you need a key to enter each corridor. It reminded me of prison back home leading me to have flashbacks. I didn't sleep all night. Next morning, I went to the charity (remember they say they are experts in supporting asylum seekers like me) and I told Roxa[7] and Amb[8] about the condition of my room and how I was having flashbacks. I asked if they could write a legal letter to get me out of there, but they told me to stay till Monday and "Man Up." I was gobsmacked, I felt so humiliated and helpless. Over the weekend I did some research in the library and wrote a letter to Home Office, myself, about the condition of the accommodation.

---

[7] Name changed for anonymity

[8] Name changed for anonymity

The response I got was an email the next day telling me they would move me to home county. I had told them the reason for my asylum, that it was causing me nightmares. Why then did they insist on treating me this way? Never have I been so humiliated. It felt like I needed the experience so that I could put that down on my CV. To say I have braved it, I survived it. When I wrote to my MP, she spoke with the Home Office saying how can you put a vulnerable person in a place that reminds them of a prison? My MP is not a trained psychologist yet she understood how the situation I was in was impacting me more than any therapist I had seen. More than any person in the Home Office.

I have never met anyone so feigned, fake, phony, pretentious, pompous as Prof Corny[9] and Dr Cruella.[10] They lied to my face, they shook my hand after we spoke. They said what they were going to do for me, to copy me in all emails, but they never did. I never received any of what we spoke about it in writing. These jokers even had the nerve to asked me why I am so peeved off. It's not rocket science or brain surgery to see why I was peeved off, who wouldn't be? Dr Cruella went one step further and hid notes from me so I wouldn't know what was on my medical report, but when I confronted her, she acted as I was deranged. She started to tell more lies, to say I was losing the plot. She started spout disinformation to my GP, saying I was becoming psychotic. But I saw my GP on a weekly basis, so she knew I was okay. She knew that being street homeless and the people at the charity treating me like shit was causing my low mood. This entire situation made me become suicidal and I tried to end my life.

---

[9] Name changed for anonymity

[10] Name changed for anonymity

It seemed the one thing Dr Cruella understood about how social stuff plays into mental health was my friends. I love and confide in my friends such as Alexandro the photography teacher who paid with her own money so I could stay in a hotel for the weekend. The yoga teacher who asked if I need any winter stuff. They treated me with dignity, saw me as a human being. They didn't stop at asking me how I was and then saying their job was done. Actions speak louder than words but this isn't something therapists are taught apparently. The therapists just use trick after trick, such bullshit to diminish my capacity. And when I try to call them out on it, I guess the truth is hard to swallow when you choking on your pride.

At this point I knew something was wrong with charity I just couldn't pin it down. They were stringing me along saying how they wanted to help but ignoring my suggestions and oppressing me, and suppressing any opportunity for help outside of them. For example, someone offered to host me in their place, but when asking the charity about me, the charity denied they even knew me. Zoey[11] the housing and welfare officer at the charity seemed to not be real. She never spoke with me directly until I kicked off and said I wasn't sure if she was real or a robot. She was so brash and rude, shouting at me for calling her.

There was another charity who wanted to give me a place, but Zoey said she didn't know me. I guess she was right how do you get to know someone? It is not that she didn't know me, she never wanted to know me. She never wanted to spend 10 minutes to get to know me. At this point I was fed up with all of them and told them to fuck off, I had enough of their mental torture.

---

[11] Name changed for anonymity

Trying to clear the air

Just before Christmas I went to try to settle the issues that the charity has created. I suggested we both meet at a neutral place like a cafe where no one feels they are superior or intimidated, but they refused. I was told by another therapist at the charity that the CEO wanted to help me. Do you get it yet? Basically, they were fucking with my mind. Gaslighting me. Saying they wanted to help and deliberately not helping. They knew what I wanted to hear and I would let my guard down. They were playing all these mind games but the easier thing to do was to give me a roof, a safe warm place.

I was trapped by them. When I told them what the mental health staff at St Thomas Hospital and other places had told me they refused to listen. They refused to talk to other therapists and people that helped me. Even my crisis case worker called Zoey to tell her that I have seen another therapist who said I was fine, but Zoey was not interested and didn't care. She is the welfare officer! I have never met such ignorant smarmy people who call themselves Experts. Experts in causing more trauma and more anxiety, maybe.

Afterall this I wanted to see my entire file. They were reluctant to give it to me so I ended up with only a quarter of it. It was full of mistakes and lies so I went straight to the CEO of the charity who had the nerve to say, "my staff can never make any mistakes." the staff were mostly white who dealt with me. From that moment I knew they were not only ignorant but racist too. They called the police to show me out, when all I was doing was asking them nicely for my own file. I even asked the charity why don't you investigate when your staff have lied and humiliated to me so much it has caused my mental health to deteriorate.

What now?

I withdrew my consent from the charity, requesting them not share information with anyone but they ignored this saying they cared. That I couldn't make an informed decision. They sent information over to my GP. My GP was so shocked by what was written. I wrote to the trustees of the charity asking them to make the staff stop harassing me, stop sending false info about me. After all they said I couldn't make an informed decision, then how come I could write to each of their trustees. How could I write calling out the errors in my notes line by line.

They were shocked like a deer caught in headlights. Why? Because when a person like me who is supposed to be an asylum seeker cam speak, read, and write English. Who is very sharp and can call them out for their lies, faults, and bullshit. I am a brown person who has no status, but I can call them out, that must have really caused a big dent in the pride and ego. They must have forgot that I was educated in America and from the streets too in America; we call a spade a spade, we don't sugar coat anything and whatever comes up we call it out.

I complained to the UKCP[12] only to find they were not interested and only cared about protecting their members. They said all of this with my file was an administrative error. But when I asked them to explain what they meant – given I had spoken to Prof Corny and Dr Cruella about getting my notes face to face, how they had promised to include me in emails but didn't? How can it be an administrative error?

All these psychotherapists have a free reign to do anything, to manipulate and play with people's lives as

---

[12] United Kingdom Council for Psychotherapists

—

44

they know they can hide behind an association. They use the police if you are more persistent in asking them to explain themselves. They get you branded as the one with issues or as the aggressor. So many people who have disdain toward the system don't speak out because nothing ever happens.

Experts in what?

After complaining about my mental health and the conditions I was living in on the street I was placed in a hotel in Ilford. I was given a social worker named OMZ[13] who was the most insensitive, ignorant person. She planned a 3-hour assessment on zoom without even considering if I had access to a device that could use zoom or enough credit for the call. These are just basic questions, who don't need a university degree to know to ask that? When I spoke with her, she got agitated when I would question her, how dare I question her. She told *'we are the ones with the qualifications'* and *'we know best.'* But I am the one with trauma. How could she invalidate me like that. She must know this will only cause me more trauma. She asked for me to consent to her contacting my GP so they increase my medication. Just like the therapists all she did was talk down to me and her answer is: have a pill for quick fix because then they don't have to listen or deal with the issue. When I called to complain about her to her manager, I was told she was new but shouldn't have said that. If she is so new, then how is she allowed to assess vulnerable people? Can they even comprehend what damage that could do to vulnerable folks?

It is so ironic to see that people of colour are overrepresented as mental health patients yet

---

[13] Name changed for anonymity

underrepresented as decision-makers in the mental health system and its governing bodies. It's like they don't trust us to know what we need or that we can make the right choice for ourselves. That is why we need some white folks to tell us what is good for us and what we need. They are just capitalising on our trauma. We are not even in charge of what treatment we want, or which treatment is best for us. It reminds the time of a master and slave - if you think culture is expensive then try ignorance. Give me nature where I am free to have the fresh air pumping in my lungs. Give me my Buddhist teachings over a pill and these 'therapist'.

It was devastating': what happened when therapy made things worse. It worsened my mental health rather than resulting in any improvement! How do you even measure the social, psychosocial, and emotional effect or the human cost of misdiagnosing someone and amplifying their traumas? They are mentally scarred and will be forever.

4

THE DEATH OF THE PERSON – Dele Oladeji

1.

Racism. Slavery. Tribalism. Imperialism. Apartheid. Survival. Death. Resurrection. Change.

Lancelot Andrews House, South London, December, 1992.

Late at night it was. I suffer from incontinence. I needed the baby nappy, you see. I couldn't survive otherwise. So I said to her, the evil Russian White Witch at Lancelot Andrews House in my desperate, tired, weak voice:

'Katharina, please, I need the nappy. I'm wetting myself. I need a nappy right now.'

She looked stunned. She has no empathy or sympathy for the homeless, the lost and wasted lives like mine. She's a witch, a very bad witch too. She's got the power; she's got the evil attitude. She's got the complete racist psychology. She's got the groove.

'I need the nappy,' said I again. 'I can't control my bladder.' She looked at me with scorn. I could feel it all. Her hatred, arrogance and disgust. She said to me aggressively as she could:

'What do you want, Black Boy?'

I said, 'I want a nappy to hold my bladder.' Somehow my own accent sounded distorted, twisted and strange.

She started laughing and sniggering then. Her colleague, a black man named Jermaine from the Caribbean Island laughed wildly too. They joked about me with intense pleasure.

'I've been given nappies in the past. Your colleague, the Irish man, Dermot does give me nappies. Give me nappies and I'll walk away,' said I.

She replied with clear pleasure and disdain:
'You Black Bastard! Why don't you return to where you came from! Go back home, pray to God like people like you do always! Praying and praying but no response from your God!'

I was lost. My confidence dropped to the bottom of my existence. This is Britain! This is South London! This is winter time in England!
'This shouldn't be happening!' I yelled. I was lost and confused. I was angry and frustrated.
I was dying with anxiety and psychosis.
She gathered her thoughts and shouted at me with authority, ruthlessness and rage:
'Fuck off! You don't belong here! Fuck off or else I'll throw you out of here!'

Jermaine was rolling around in laughter. He thought it was some kind of joke. I became a laughing stock for the evening. Then he, a tall, huge black man with a South London accent opened the huge black door, dragged me on the floor and threw me out into the evening chill. I felt prejudice. I felt racism. He yelled loudly at me before slamming the door:
'Fuck off now and return to the jungle! That's where you belong!'

He was laughing and chuckling all the way through. I thought he'd be on my side, being a black man himself. But that wasn't the case. It was fun time for him, kicking me and yelling. Witch Katharina was like that too in unison, laughing and chuckling. Just laughing to her heart's content. It was a dark memorable day I'll never forget: buried deep in my mentality, layered in racism.

They don't even know my name. They refuse to know my name.

2.

The chill of the winter months got me wandering. My helpless, wasted self along the cold, busy London streets, journeying through the dark times, the vileness that goes with homelessness, racism, mental illness. And all the time my thoughts wandering also: my unclear understanding of myself and where I belong in society.

My mental health was very frail. I needed my damn medication.
What a wasted human entity with no class or status!

Randy Crawford started playing around in my musing mind. *Rainy Night in Georgia* was the song. Then the cold night got colder and colder. I was freezing very badly. I weed myself on the spot, shivering terribly from the cold, chilly night. It started to rain notoriously and heavily.
Schizophrenia! The bastard of madnesses!

The evil voices were singing in my head. The angry voices became louder and louder. Lancelot Andrews House! That abode for wasted souls. Those forgotten, dark, troubled voices. All those wasted human entities begging and crying.

I died within. I couldn't rise up to fight my corner or express my thoughts or feelings. I felt tormented, shredded and separated from society and existence. I wanted God badly but I couldn't find God. I wanted hope terribly but I couldn't find hope.

My self-esteem and confidence had dropped drastically to the bottom of life: It felt like I had disappeared into space, surrounded by inequality, oppression and discriminated against within the strands of humanity, dirt and survival. Racism was eating me up very badly. My guts got twisted and knotted. My teary brown eyes were raging with madness, anger and suicidal thoughts. My voice became weaker and weaker. My hearing travelled further from the sounds of the city.

This was the beginning, the death of me. Again, I heard raging dark, hopeless voices in my weary head. They weren't happy voices.

Through the hue of the murky window, I could see and hear Katharina's stern voice. Distant but clear in my head. I could see her deep-set blue eyes. Jermaine's husky voice was ringing clearly too.

'You loony bin,' she was saying through the open window. 'Return to Africa and pray to God like you always do. There's no room for you here.'
A range of laughter was all I could hear. Their laughter! Laughter! More Laughter!

Pain and Denial. Darkness. Homelessness. Prejudice. Anguish. Voices. Racism. Segregation.

But I turned a different corner. I could see the distant road ahead of me. The road was long. I couldn't see beyond a certain point of view. Still:
Madness! Pain! Rage! Anguish! Death!

3.

Another journey started. Into a newly found society.

I was voyaging into the realms of the fairy angels. The kind angels, the lovely angels singing in the Garden of Eden.
The evil snake that changed the outlook of the universe with its hiss.

The image of Eve appeared like I was in a deep trance.

The new start in life beckoned and moved me on. I wanted to be stable, strong, and boldly drive myself towards stability but racism lingered in the air:
The Metropolitan Police Service, London! A newly found passion awaited me: policing our diverse city. Living on the edge of passion and being a genius.

A new dream started but not for long…
Who was I? Who am I? Am I racist too? Am I going to die? Will I ever stand tall to fight my corner?

What a fresh start this seemed to be after all the years of homelessness, racism and mental illness. I thought I was in a different world, a beautiful world. Working in a very busy custody suite in London. I thought I had it all to myself.

Oh, what a dream. I dreamed I had it all! Was I correct in my judgement? No, I wasn't. The torment started all over again.

The past dreams and the new world collided.

There were no differences. I wanted to work hard and give back to society. I wanted my own dreams and aspirations. I wanted recovery and success. I wanted stability and inclusion.

I wanted a world far away from racism, slavery and oppression. But it's all there, running around within our varied worlds.

Oppression! Madness! Pain and Racism! Tribalism! Segregation and Prejudice! Hopelessness!

4.

I returned back in time. I always dream back to Lancelot Andrews House.

The evil shone again on the horizon. I remember those days very well: all the vileness and addictions playing the game all around me once again. Marijuana it was, crack cocaine, speed, Chasing the Dragon, skunk, alcoholism and drunkenness racing to win. I had to exist somehow.

Drinking cans of Special Brew at night along the quiet, lonesome streets that buzzed and were buried with hidden lives, trashiness and excitements. Smoking cigarettes and tobacco, burning madly inside out like an overworked old chimney that erupts on a cold winter evening. Downing litres of cider to get rid of the pain and anguish.

It was all in the madness trip to hell! A journey towards Satan in his secluded, ferocious den. Death calling out like the sounds of a wild rock and roll band on a wild night, playing the dark music game. The anger game. The madness game. The racist game. The addiction game. The prejudice game.

Then my thoughts returning to another world: The world of policing. Metropolitan Police Service, 2005. The best police force in the whole world. The past hideous life hidden somewhere behind me:
'You, Monkey,' said he, a fresh police officer out of training school on night duty.
'Go back home, monkey. This is our country. This is my country.'
'What did you say just now, Officer Fork-Berry? What did you say?' I said.
'You bloody monkey,' he said confidently and forcefully. 'Go back home! Go back!'

'But what are you trying to say? That you're better than me?'

'Only a joke, matey,' he said. 'Only a joke! Don't take it personal. It's all a game. Be happy, man! You need to learn the game to understand the game! It's not personal,' he said.

Then he and his mate, Officer Junky started laughing.

'He's taking it personal,' he said. 'This is our world now, monkey. If you can't adapt, fuck off!'

The joke went further into the deep dark lonely night.

He couldn't stop doing the monkey impersonation. Dancing around like he was hanging from a tree or jumping about like a wild beast.

'You're black anyway, aren't you?' he said.

'Does it really matter?' said I.

I was floating in denial, anger and rage. I had to stand tall. I had to stay bold and brave and just carry on living and surviving. I had to fight my own wars, my own battles.

I was in and out of time, back and forth with time.

'It shouldn't be the case, Sergeant Forrester,' I said when I reported the incident of bullying and racism. 'Why was he doing the monkey moves when there was a black man around? What was he trying to say to me, to you, to us?'

'Matey, forget about it. You won't go far in the job if you take this matter further. This is the Met! The best police force in the world! If you don't like the way you were treated, hand in your warrant card and head off home. Now, fuck off! Is that alright, officer? Fuck off, now. Go on the dole,' he said. 'It's there for people like you.'

My world collapsed. I really liked the Met. I wanted to work there and stay for as long as I could but I was wrong. In modern times, that kind of racist attitude is unwarranted! Un-forgivable!

5.

Then I moved back again. My life fell apart; I wanted to work hard to find sanity, recovery and stability. But my psychosis cried. My madness heightened drastically.

The daily angry voices were in my head, bashing, yelling and crying. Singing and dancing. Loving, crying and hating, buried within the multi-colours of hatred and anguish. Why should my world be one of isolation and loneliness? The drugs and alcohol don't work. They make matters worse.

The situation became darker and darker like the darkness encountered en-route to hell. The colours of the world changed senselessly through the guided barricades of shattered hopes and dreams.

Hell became a home in my head. Dreaming a nice space in hell. Racism ringing my bells to the universe. The voice of God disappeared. The fairy angels drifted away too.

Madness! Racism! Prejudice! Hatred!

I aren't who I was anymore. My spirituality ran away from me.

Darkness! Pain! Rage! Frustration!

Racism kept ruling the world we live in, in varied strands, and aspects of life, like mine, evident in the work environment. In the carrying out of my daily activities. In our confused politics, in our diverse societies and the world that failed to connect with us existentially. In our inter-marriages. In what we believe to be right from wrong. In what made us question ourselves far away from oppression, prejudice and racism. It was there, it still existed, buried deep beneath the corners of our minds, our survival.

Racism kept flashing in my imagination, in the manner in which I connected with people: my sheer disbelief about social endeavours and my intense truthfulness and appreciation of life that got knocked down by the colours and presence of racism that I felt. I kept trying to move forward with life. But there was confusion and dirt, denial, pain, anger and hopelessness. There was prejudice roaming around aimlessly in my trajectory.

Imperialism! Angry voices! Happy voices! Prejudice! Dreaming to God!

I started dreaming all over again with no sense of direction. I dreamed my entire world, my universe, my own lone planet. I imagined a new world, a changed society.

The resurrection of the dead, the wasted person that's fighting for life, survival, hope and peace. The strength, pride and resilience of the person that shines and hopes for a brighter world; a universal world! This person is the creator, the protector and the survivor. The people in this context were those that struggled to find their unique voices.

I wanted to listen to the unheard voices of the common people and voices of positivity:

The colour of racism was drifting away. The young generation were creating a new society for us. No more drinking cheap cider in the hidden street corners! I need no more nappies! No more shitting myself! No more anger, rage or hatred in my troubled life. No more suicidal thoughts in the head. No more racism in any shape, colour or form. Pain is gone. Today's society is receptive of cultures, beliefs, religion and political aspirations. The world we live in now is powerful, showing a united society, a critical political sphere, a unique world that fights and sings against racism and accepting democracy and a universal mode of existence for peoples within places and beyond.

But in today's world I journeyed along the long, dark, endless road into the abyss.

The road was long and thirsty for death. The road was dangerous and hopeless. I wanted to grieve for my mental ill-health but racism, prejudice and segregation kept running after me everywhere I went.

Who in this world is my anchor!? Will my skin colour be a question for political debate?

6.

Again, I went back to Lancelot Andrews House. It was a strange, worthless day with Bully Robson, the skinhead from Burton-On-Trent who found himself homeless and living rough in the very busy streets of London. Mental ill-health, racism and homelessness layered in a human cocoon of darkness and isolation. So he spoke to me angrily on a very slow nighty-night. I was already dreaming a new bright day ahead of me. It was 10 in the evening. He said to me with extreme hatred, excitement and precision:

'Speedy, dance for me or I'll smash in your hopeless black head. Dance for me like the black hopeless bitch you are!'

'But I'm not a dancer, Robson. I ain't a dancer. I truly can't dance, Rob. I can't…'

'Ha, the black bitch doesn't want to dance this evening. He's having an episode this evening. He is wetting his pants again this evening. Oh, he's hearing voices in his drugged up head this evening. Dance for me, Speedy!

Dance for me or else I'll smash your freaky head in!' He puffed around. He was irate. Very irate.

'I can't. Please, I can't dance. Let me be, I can't dance!'

'Do the fucking moves, bitch, or else I'll smash your...' He'd lost his last words. He looked intensely into my dying eyes and spat his thick saliva in my face.

Everyone present started laughing. The whole world was laughing at me. I had no power, no status; no class. It was me and Robson. He's a short man with loads of tattoos on his pale face and body. He's heavily built and limps on one foot. No hair on his head. He's got silver rings on every finger on his hands.

Somehow, I started to dance. No one to protect me. It was that fearful and that hopeless. It was a recipe for the angry voices in my head. God had drifted away. Lucifer wasn't miles away either, very happy and gay. How do I deal with this level of racism and dirt and filth and pain and drug use and alcoholism and loneliness and prejudice and craziness? How do I navigate these hordes of angry thoughts and filth that kept running after me every single day, every single hour, every single minute and every single second? Adam and Eve created these darknesses for us to live with. God has also discharged us from his careful, tolerant watch. Satan was now in charge of our hectic, hopeless world.

My life was under the canopy of death. I was hoping and waiting. I was waiting in vain. Waiting and waiting and waiting. Racism had turned my head upside down. I wanted peace, hope and stability. Homelessness shredded my guts, my brain and my physical well-being, in and out of space.

I was floating high in the blue skies, dreaming a new beginning.

7.

Inspector Rackety couldn't come up with the recipe for change and a new world. He blamed it all on the existence of religion and searching for God. The God that never shows his face.

'People like you believe in God too much,' he said.

Inspector Rackety was a pretender. He thought he was the big deal in the force. He placed himself so high no one could reach him. He was wrong and I was right. He said to me:

'I know your father passed away, PADDA, and you need some time off.'

'Yes, Gov,' I said. 'My father has passed. May I get some time off? Gov, my father's gone.'

'So who's going to do the bloody work then?' he said.

'But sir, I need more time off! My father has passed on. I need time off.'

'If you can't accept a few days off, then fuck off and get out of here! I'm the King!' he said.

'But Mr. Rackety, just let me win for once. I need more time off.'

Everything changed after that encounter.
I thought I was in a safe place. I thought I'd be protected and supported. I rarely talked about my mental health because I felt I'd be judged for it. But racism heightened my madness and propelled me further into isolation and loneliness.

Why am I still on this planet? Where was God when I needed him most?

Where were the psychiatrists, the psychologists, and other clinicians when I needed them most? The entire town was laughing at me now.

Darkness! Voices! Madness! Pain and Anguish! Passion! Hope! Prejudice! Law and Order! The Media and our

Existence! Politics and Power! Sexuality! Culture! Empathy! Death! Medication, Cure and Recovery!

Lancelot Andrews House, South London, 1992. Then arose Spur House, South London, 1993. Spur House, the den of iniquity. The darkly home for the lost and forgotten voices.

8.

Dinner time!

'Come queue for your meals,' shouted Bobby, the tall, lanky English white chef in charge of the kitchen. There was a level of hierarchy in the dining room at Spur House. The loved ones got the best part of the daily sloppy meals. The rest of the gang had to live with whatever they were given. So I being a young black man, it became difficult to connect and understand the 'status theory' that dictated how we lived. The politics at Spur House were greater than the power tussle between politicians and governance. The politics were based on racism, prejudice and class. A world of hatred and all that goes with power, status and hierarchy. Bobby was the leader of all this vileness.

'Yes, that's your portion this evening,' he said to Roaming Davido.

'Yes, that's your portion,' he said to Jolly Paul.

'Yes, that's your portion,' he said to Jimmy.

'Yes, that's your portion,' he said to Scottish Dave.

'That's your portion,' he said to Remy.

'Yes, that's your portion,' he said lovingly to Ricardo.

'And that's yours and yours and yours and yours and yours too,' he said to Eddie, Bruno, Charlie, Tanji and Lawrence. 'And yours and yours,' said he to George and Frankie.

'And yours too! Yes, yours, that's your portion!' he said to Wild, Cunning Richard.

'And yours,' he said to Simple Minded Lucky-Boy! 'And yours!' said he warmly to Crazy Rory. 'And yours' to Funny Edmond.

'And yours…' He paused awhile.

'And yours, let me think…And yours… Wait and die,' he said angrily.

'Yes,' he said. 'None of this is for you, African Bloody Twat. Go back to the end of the queue and start all over again. Yours will come once everyone else's been served.'

I tried to fight my corner with the little strength left within. I thought I could fight my corner but I couldn't make it happen as I wished. I had to stay hungry sometimes because of fear of being called silly names like Speedy, like the Black Bitch, like the Michelin Man, like the African Bloody Twat! Like the Bitch needing baby nappies. Like the Hover that scoops up everything. Like the Evil, Black Bitch that enjoys drinking Special Brew and likes smoking weed and tobacco.

In my true colour none of these made sense. I created an image of a protector in my head. Hurst! Sweet, sweet, Dear happy, Hurst; my guardian, my saviour, my friend, my protector.

Hurst, the imaginary white spirit that sings to me in my heavy head. Hurst, the living being that distracts racist voices in my psyche. Hurst, the spiritual entity that prays for me and guides me all the time. Hurst, the mad, happy, jolly being that reads to me and gets me grounded.

This was the death of the person but we do not want the death of the person. Life can be tastily sweet, overwhelming pleasurable and challenging but racism is a silent villain that separates and creates chaos and unhappiness in our demanding world. Racism is not sweet but vile, hopeless and evil. It's not the death of the person here now, but the future of the person that's living and existing. It's not the death of the person, no, it's not the death of the person at all. Death in itself is nothing to humankind but the shadow of our existences. I'll stand tall! I'll fight my corner, and I'll conquer the planet! I'll keep fighting against racism for as long as I live.

I'm glad that Katharina and Jermaine kicked me out of the hostel. That truly made me a better version of myself, crying out loud against racism, prejudice and homelessness.

I'll keep on fighting my corner to the utmost point of my wasted, troubled life. I'll celebrate my existence in style and hopefulness. I will survive, my lovely, jolly friends. I'll live and survive in this changeable, formidable universe! Peace!

STORIES OF RACISM IN MENTAL HEALTH SERVICES

5

AM I COMPLICIT IN THE RACIALISED EXPERIENCE OF THE MENTAL HEALTH SYSTEM? A CARER'S PERSPECTIVE – Cassandra Lovelock

Introduction

Being a Black service user in UK mental health services means being coerced, silenced and ignored. Being Black mixed-race in UK mental health services means being subject to some quick colourism maths, then being coerced, silenced and ignored. As a carer trying to enact your rights to be part of the care team, you're seen as a nuisance, you're ignored. My complexion, bone structure and figure seem to entitle statutory services to push blame on me. Blame my culture for not knowing the risks; assume English is not my first language so they should not even try explaining things to me. Decide that my home environment is a bad place for my sister's recovery because it must be so vastly different.

My sister was severely mentally ill for most of the memories I have of her. A lot of those involve statutory mental health settings and persons and their overbearing presence in our lives. As a young teenager, I stepped up to support her in the only ways you know how to as a teenager – which to be honest was not that many. But I took the time to learn, educate myself and be 'educated' by mental health services. In this learning, I no doubt internalised the racism the mental health system is built upon, and acted based upon that system until I was at a point where I realised, I was allowed to question it.

In some ways writing here about racism in mental health services feels like preaching to a devoted choir, but this piece of writing is both a thought piece and a confession. Was I, as a young carer, a teenage carer and then an adult carer, was I complicit in the racist system? How did this impact my relationship with my sister? Second-hand experiences of racism in the mental health system can be traumatic – but can I claim to be traumatised by this racism? Or do I just have a guilty conscience?

Why did viewing what was obviously racist practice not radicalise and turn me against the mental health system sooner? Why did I continue to trust the system's decisions up until some would argue it was too late? My sister died in November 2016 by suicide. She'd been released from a PICU two days before and no one told me.

Breaking the Trust

I'm 13 and my sister is screaming. Being restrained by four mental health nurses, one of which has their knee digging into her neck. They are holding her down cause visiting time is over and I am leaving, they are blaming me for her 'violent outburst.'

Trusting mental health services was never posed as a decision. Merely as a 9-year-old you trusted the structures you grew up in. We are taught from a young age to trust the health system. Ring an ambulance when something is wrong with your body, and they'll help. Ring the police when something has happened that threatens your safety, and they'll help. At what age can ignorance no longer be accepted as a justification?

—

64

I didn't know this was not how she should have been treated; that they were using excessive force. I didn't know I wasn't to blame for her behaviour; I thought I was because they told me so. I thought I shouldn't visit because my attendance caused her distress – an odd thing to realise as the white family also visiting their loved one leaves without being yelled at for their presence.

I'm 16 and a person on the ward my sister is on has cornered me yelling racial abuse. They call me the 'n' word, they call me a Black bitch. I find my sister and she is scrubbing at her skin, begging to whatever she is seeing to make her white. To make the person stop terrorising her.

Taking the blame for decisions statutory services make is the defining experience of being a caregiver, and as a child, I did not know any better. When my sister was racially abused while on a mixed ward, my conversation about it with her 'increased her sensitivity'. When this racial abuse led to self-harm and skin scrubbing, when she begged for discharge, I told her to stay. I agreed with her care team this was the best place for her – yes, because I did not have the 'capacity' to keep her safe at home – but this was clearly not a safe environment for her. Despite asking her care team to transfer her to another ward, or ideally move the perpetrator, I was met with the same blame and victim blaming: 'she's not actually Black, why is she reacting so badly' and '[perpetrator] isn't saying anything that bad, we'll give her Midazolam.' This was coupled with their own defensiveness – how they were taking care of her for me, how I should be grateful.

Patient-to-patient racism is missing from academic literature, grey literature, policy or guidelines.

I could google as much as I liked but there was nowhere to go to get this situation changed besides discharge. Who are you meant to complain to? How was I meant to advocate for my sister's needs when every IMHA she had was a white person? Who is in the position to illustrate that a patient being racist to another patient isn't part of their illness, it's their bigotry and hated? Bigotry that saw my sister being picked on: being viewed as an easier target due to being female, a less intimidating, less aggressive target as a mixed-race person than the Black men and woman also on the ward. It was the perpetrator's bigotry that my sister paid the price for, and I dealt with those consequences. And just like that, the trust - which was never built up - was shattered.

Coerced into Coercion

I'm 17 and arguing against my sister being given a CTO. I'm begging this mental health social worker, telling them that these drugs won't help – and having police escort to inject them won't either.

Keating et al (2002)[14] found in their report 'Breaking the Circles of Fear' that Black people have a strong and profound mistrust of services, resisting seeking help and thus presenting only at crisis.

Despite the claims made by psychiatry to be evidenced-based, when presented with people who respond to distress in ways that subvert the norm, instead of seeking knowledge from those that may be equipped with it, statutory mental health services panic.

This is how my sister ended up with a Community Treatment Order (CTO) coupled with a curfew and regular

---

14

**https://www.centreformentalhealth.org.uk/sites/default/files/
publication/download/breaking_the_circles_of_fear.pdf**

---

drug testing. At this point I would like to remind you all –
she was not a criminal.

*I'm 17 and one cop is threatening my sister's arrest if she
doesn't accept this jab. The other tells me to buck up. That
it's better she is forced to take these drugs and sleep 20
hours a day and scream the other four than be my sister.
For the first time I ask if they are doing this to other people
too and they say only the bad ones.*

Community Treatment Orders are a common experience
for Black people enrolled within the mental health system;
they are a technique used to ensure compliance with
treatment. They are advertised as an effective way to keep
a service user out of hospital and in the community; in
reality, they are a method of removing free will. People
under a CTO can be held to curfews and drug-testing,
being unable to leave certain areas. If at any point, the
clinicians are unhappy with the service user, they can be
re-called to hospital. If the service user refuses
medication, they are returned to hospital; if they socialise
with the 'wrong people', they are returned to hospital.

If you are a carer, a CTO causes your level of
responsibility for the service user to increase significantly.
Carers are coerced into being the enforcer; sometimes
they have no choice but to be the enforcer. My sister's
practitioners forced me to compel her into treatment using
my love as both the bait and bully. I hated letting them in
the house, I hated begging my sister to not run upstairs;
watching them chase her. I hated the feeling of
powerlessness as the nurse injected medication into my
sister, hated listening to her cry and beg for them not to do
it. I hate being threatened with section 135, watching them
dangle it in front of me if I didn't comply and let all this
happen.

Let us in or we can force our way. Let's do this the easy way. We'll be back with a 135 warrant if you don't so open the door. You can't afford to replace it after all.

I hated being the one to guilt trip her into accepting her medication, desperate to keep her at home and terrified for her to be there at the same time. In this experience I wonder if, indeed, I am complicit in this racist practice, if, if, if.

An Apology

I'm 15 and my sister is crying. They've cut her hair cause her afro is 'too difficult to manage.' I don't understand.

While there is little causal evidence that racism within the mental health systems was a destructive force within my sister's and my relationship, I cannot ignore the correlation. The tensions from CTO orders and my inability to defend/advocate for my sister's needs had profound impacts on our relationship and other interpersonal relationships.

I appreciate this essay positions mental health treatment as a Them and Us narrative, which it certainly is not and should never be. With that being said:

I didn't know I needed to defend her against the racism of the system, I didn't know experiencing racism was traumatising. I couldn't reconcile how the places I was told would keep you safe were hurting you, were causing you harm.

I didn't know how to challenge a system that was also treating me in awful ways, that was exploiting both my naivety and my love for you. I was a teenager and I didn't have the language to argue with your care team, I didn't have the power, my knowledge wasn't good enough, applied enough, was not the right type of expert. I didn't have the qualifications, the reputation, the social standing, or the time.

I didn't know being critical of psychiatry was allowed. There wasn't an end game or a singular event that made me critical of mental health services. There is no way to see mental health services as a separate system when they build upon and allow abuse from other institutions including the police and social care services.

I was pushed to enact their racist practices and whether it came from love or from wanting my sister home and not in hospital, I cannot act like I am innocent in this mess. I was caught in the dual roles of caring endlessly but being the custodian. Of enforcing their racism. Breaking her trust again and again as she was in another inpatient unit, in another city, another promise that this one would be better, that she'd be safer there. And these racist structures, this racism is what destroyed my sister's and my relationship. Whether or not I had a hand in a racist incident, in the end I was to blame because I did not try hard enough to prevent it.

I'm sorry. I love you. As with everything, this is for you.

6

HOW CAN I REASON OR BEGIN TO MAKE SOMEONE UNDERSTAND? – A. Peony

There had been a long gap since I had seen a psychologist at my CMHT as the one I had been working with left. We had just started making headway as at the time I was experiencing an influx of flashbacks from traumatic events in my life. This was the first time Complex Post-Traumatic Stress Disorder (CPTSD) had been brought up in my sessions and I was struggling to cope. I felt stuck in a shell. It was also the first time I had really truly acknowledged any trauma, and the years of it all surfaced up at once.

I had no coping strategies or idea where to begin, so when the psychologist I was working with suddenly left after just a few sessions of focusing on trauma, I was taken aback and worried about if I could manage alone. Before she left, she had arranged for me to meet another psychologist, but this would be whenever there was availability. It was quite a bit of a gap in time till I met this new psychologist, and when the time came, I felt somewhat hopeful I would finally get some help to work through CPTSD. However, my first session was focused on the "D" word - she was focused on Discharging me from psychological services and said that her impression was this session was just to check in and discharge. I was very confused as that was not what I was told. There was a back and forth, and ultimately she agreed to see me again as she said she didn't want to force a discharge, but at the same time I did not get the impression she wanted to continue sessions with me.

There was again a lot of back and forth in the sessions, where she would counter anything I said. There was a disconnection between the two of us, a clear distinction between class, social, cultural background and me being a person of colour. As I continued sessions with her, this became more and more apparent and affected the therapy/treatment, her assumptions about me, my situation and later on, her would-be diagnosis. Her emphasis and focus were on what she saw me as: someone who was distrustful and troubled. I thought I would be getting support with post-traumatic stress as it was really taking its toll on me and trickling into all parts of my life, but there wasn't much focus on this nor the severity of the situation.

A Battle to Be Heard

Being from my close-knit community, full of different generations where most people know each other and live in close proximity, including extended family members and friends of family and so on, it is hard to have privacy. On some level, everyone knows or knows of one another, and this means people often share and talk about others. After sessions, mental health reports/care plans are sent back to my GP surgery, and they would often go missing there. The receptionists and patient management staff are from my community, and also have access to these patient files and notes. I was always worried to hear that my private notes were lying around somewhere in the surgery when they would say they couldn't find them. Whenever I tried to explain this, the psychologist would dismiss me and just reiterate the same thing about privacy laws, which I am familiar with, but that doesn't mean that people/professionals actually follow protocol.

The psychologist often wanted me to share information I did not feel comfortable to share with her. Firstly, because we didn't have a good rapport, and I was also just coming to terms with my traumatic experiences. These were things that happened that I had never said out loud, things I didn't even have the words to say. I was struggling with reliving these traumatic flashbacks; I was in no place to share details. Nor did I feel like I was in a safe space to open up. I didn't feel assured of my privacy, especially with reports and care plans going missing. It bothered me as it's sensitive, private information, especially if mental health professionals are asking me and noting down the details of my traumatic experiences.

These sessions with her made me feel as though she saw me as a very paranoid person whose distrust was misplaced. She would not open herself up to my view, as a brown person living in community. The dismissal of my lived experience and experiences of friends and family I know too, hurt and confused me. Even more so as whenever this came up, I would always acknowledge that if I was not in this tight-knit community, I wouldn't question my privacy. Objectively it makes no sense for her to discount my experience as she has no experience of living in a brown body in my social and cultural community. What is interesting, is that I have revisited this issue with other mental health professionals who happened to be of similar background to me; I found they did not discount my experience and reasoning behind this, nor was it something I had to go over repeatedly.

Something is Always Lost in Translation

What made it worse was that it seemed she was oblivious to her prejudice and how this prejudice made her react and treat me as a patient with discrimination and bias.
I dreaded my appointments but felt I had to keep going as it was better than nothing, and I didn't want to seem like I wasn't complying or trying. I didn't feel like I got anything out of those sessions apart from leaving each one feeling bad about myself, even questioning myself. It felt like a

battle of trying to be heard and seen but instead she left me feeling like I was over-exaggerating. Now I realise I was just being gaslighted. I had years of trauma resurfacing and ultimately I just wanted some help and support to get through what happened to me over the years, and I didn't get that. Instead, it felt like each session I was being questioned and made to feel like I was making a big thing out of nothing.

On top of this, she so readily encouraged me to tell my family about the trauma I experienced over the years. I felt like we were going round in circles. She reacted as if me being uncomfortable and un-ready to open up to my family about years of trauma was misplaced. I would always feel like I was repeating myself, explaining my background and how it isn't so easy to open up like that, especially as it's a sensitive subject. She didn't understand that there would be a translation issue too – and that communication issues are a recipe for giving more trauma. When I would explain the reason why it was difficult to follow her suggestions because of my ethnic and cultural background, she dismissed me as if what I was saying wasn't true, almost as if I was making up excuses.

How can I reason or begin to make someone understand my barriers and difficulties if they refuse to acknowledge my ethnicity and my cultural and societal norms? My family is multi-generational.

My grandparent is a big part of my life and is from a much older generation. I had a lot of struggles with that during that period and the psychologist would not see that as an issue as if I was purposely making the situation more difficult than it seemed. At that time my grandparent and some family members didn't truly understand what struggling with mental health and post-traumatic stress disorder is like, for example. I am not saying that they were not supportive – even with little understanding, they were there for me in the best ways they knew how and, in my community, doors are opening for dialogue when it comes to mental health and trauma but at different speeds.

How my Brown Body is Erased

I had no idea that she had diagnosed me. Also, that was the first time I had heard of a psychologist diagnosing as that would always be the role my psychiatrist had. She had diagnosed me with Emotionally Unstable Personality Disorder (EUPD). A lot of time had passed when I noticed this diagnosis. I had stopped seeing her at that point and was with working with someone specialising in trauma.

I was confused as I didn't fit the criteria of EUPD. I even asked the new psychologist who I'd been working with for some time and she also agreed I do not fit the criteria. I had been misdiagnosed based on someone's discriminative, racist, one-sided point of view. This diagnosis of EUPD stayed on my records and has affected my getting help and treatment with physical illness.

I wonder if mental health professionals really take into consideration their words and diagnosis that imprint on our records, our patient files, our lives. The power they have and how it can have a detrimental effect. The sad thing is I don't think she'll ever realise the power of her words and her ability to place a diagnosis on me and how it's affected me going forwards.

Ultimately going to these sessions with the psychologist was supposed to be a place for support and understanding, but it just made me feel terrible. The last several sessions before I stopped seeing her made me feel worse, more anxious and the outcome was even worse. I think now looking back she did gaslight me, to a point where it was working on an insidious level that I started questioning myself and didn't get the help I needed. She erased and ignored who I am and my experiences living in this brown body. My experiences were met with being questioned or disbelieved. She didn't just make assumptions about my background; she ignored it completely.

Towards the end of our sessions together, I did bring a family member in with me because I wasn't getting anywhere and didn't feel heard. I had reached my lowest point. My family member also shared my frustration after being in that session and could see what I had been experiencing. At the end of it, the psychologist ended the topic with asking me if I ever had been an inpatient in mental health care. I realised where this was going and her intentions.

Ultimately I was struggling because of CPTSD, which trickled into all parts of my life and made other aspects of my mental health worse; I just needed the right support. But I was never going to get this support from her as she treated me as if I over-dramatised and exaggerated everything.

What I brought to the sessions didn't fit in with her dominant culture perspective, which was based in whiteness and racism. I believe my experience during this period of life would not have been this distressful if the mental health professional was not discriminative. I don't think I would have had to spend years fighting a misdiagnosis, dismissal, or as much distress. I think many of us get stuck in the fuckery that is the system. And staying there means subjecting yourself to racism in order to survive, whether economically and to make ends meet (never mind living some sort of a life), or to access mental health support. Much harm has been done over the years to those of us in the system which could have been avoided.

THE COMMUNITY MENTAL HEALTH TEAM REVIEW –
Mikloth Bond

The reason why I have asked you to this meeting, is to introduce you all to one another. First to Dr Elaine Arnold, who I have invited as an expert witness, due to her work as a psychiatric social worker and her extensive work in the field of attachment theory since 1998. Then there is Michael Houston, my church minister and the minister of Bethnal Green Mission Church. Also, Dwight Bond, my son, and probably the person here who knows me the most intimately. You are the ones who have to pick up the pieces and worry the most about me when I am unwell. So, I would like to give you all collective authority over me. I've put this in writing so that if any of you feel I am showing signs of becoming unwell and I am not responding to your requests to get medical help, I give you permission to act on my behalf, and, if necessary, have me sectioned.

I hope to have you review two things today. Firstly, whether my diagnosis is correct, and secondly if you think it is safe to reduce my medication with the view to taking me off them altogether.

You have all received my submissions I sent you in which I hope to make my case that my diagnosis should not be one of Paranoid Schizophrenia but one of lack of attachment, and I hope you have all had the chance to read them.

First of all, I would like to read you a piece I wrote last year between 24 October and 7 November, while I was attending a course at the Central and North West London Recovery and Wellbeing College. The course was called

Telling My Story, and we were asked to write a piece on 'Beginnings.'

Beginnings.

My beginning was also my end.

I refer to the day I left Guyana for England at the age of seven. My dad and mum had already left Guyana to make a life for themselves in England when I was one and two years old, respectively. So, I was brought up in Guyana by my grandmother, with my three sisters. Two of my sisters were older than me and they left to be united with my parents the year before, leaving me and my younger sister behind. Then came the day, a year later, when we were going to join our parents. We were very excited, and looking forward to finally meeting them. However just as the boat was about to pull out of port, I remember looking at my grandmother on shore, and it dawned on me that I would never see her again. I began to cry uncontrollably and would have jumped off the boat to be with her if I had not been restrained. It was a very traumatic experience, and one which I have only become aware of again recently. When we arrived in England, there was no attachment between myself and my parents. I would later say that it was the beginning of my mental health problems.

This was written at least three months before I had ever heard of attachment theory. It was not until February this year that I heard about attachment, and since then I have tried to find out as much as I can about it and how it has affected me.

I also believe that there is something else going on with me besides attachment, and that is that I might be somewhere on the autism spectrum. I first became suspicious about this thirteen years ago in 2005 after I saw a programme on TV. I approached my GP at the time, who did not take me seriously, and to tell the truth, neither did I take me seriously. As a result, a diagnosis was never pursued. However, this has come up again through different circumstances, and I have been in touch with my GP once again to have it investigated. I believe you have had a letter from my GP explaining my reasons.

I know that if you were to agree with me about the attachment issue and/or the autism that does not mean that you would necessarily believe that my diagnosis is wrong, as I believe you can have attachment issues, and autism, and still have a diagnosis of schizophrenia.
My problem is I do not know what the criteria are for a diagnosis for Paranoid Schizophrenia, and I hope you will take the time to explain to me what these are. I would also like to ask if it is possible to give me a copy of my psychiatric medical history.

In the past I have not had the cognitive capacity to deal with these issues, due to the pressures of holding down a job, and my lack of understanding of life. By this I mean that life as a way of tripping us up if we do not have the right structures to support us through the dark times and the pressures we all encounter on our journeys; structures like work, family, education, and in my case, church. But I am in quite a different place now, after my 'Great Awakening', that was when I became aware of my place in society and a way of moving forwards. This took place on 5th May 2016. Although I did initially deteriorate quite badly after my experience, I have subsequently rallied and become more connected to the people around me and to society. This experience, which may not have looked good at first, has turned out to be the reason for my seeking rehabilitation (Recovery).

Which brings me to the second part of my review: Why I would like to be taken off of my medication. Contrary to opinion, I do not now nor ever have had a problem with taking medication. However, when I am compliant in taking it, I feel that it is supposed that everything is okay: 'He is well. That's it. Job done. We need look no further.' And though we do from time to time have these reviews, the expectations of you getting to know me, or I you, are very limited.

No effort is made to rehabilitate me, and as long as I continue to take my medication, and do not raise my voice, everyone is happy. All except me. To this I am sure you will say 'But when you take your medication, you do not become ill.' However, I would dispute that. Though I do keep well for a time, I do eventually become ill again. Take, for instance the period between 1995 and 2005: I remained well for all that period then suddenly I became ill, and to date we still do not know why this was. The perceived opinion is that I stop taking my medication and so become unwell when actually, it is the other way around: I become unwell and so stop taking my medication.

So, despite being well, on my injections since September 2016, I feel that if I were to stop taking my medication, I would not become ill again.

So, why should you agree to this? I think that this is the time to try something different. Those who know me well, know that I have changed in the last 18 months, being able to reason and pursue different areas in my life in a rational way. That is why I have asked you all to be involved in my care: in order that you will be able to map my progress and bear witness to my development. I have given you power over me, so that should you feel I am becoming a danger to myself or to others, you will be able to take preventative measures. I think my rehabilitation is progressing well, but I still feel caged by my history. I feel that this would be the right time, under strict control, and observation, to try, if it is okay with you, to unlock that cage.

I put these two reviews to you in the hope that you will help me understand more fully where you are coming from. Also for you to know the things that worry me and prevent me from moving on. I so much want to have a good relationship with you, and be involved in working out how to achieve the best result in integrating me fully into society, and at the same time developing me into the best me that I can be.

Mikloth Bond - April 2018

Since my CMHT Review

I had quite a struggle persuading the psychiatrist at my review to allow me to read the above statement, and after I had done so, his remarks were: 'We don't do rehabilitation. That is not what this service is about.'
Though I was surprised to hear this, I was not too disappointed as I had already discovered the Recovery College, which offers rehabilitation through Recovery principles. Those principles are: Your recovery should be self-directed; your path is based on personal needs, likes, and experience; your recovery should empower you; and your recovery should include your mental, physical and spiritual needs.

The Recovery College is an NHS organisation that offers courses for people with mental health issues, as well as for mental health professionals, along with carers. All the courses are co-produced, which means an expert by experience (on mental health) working alongside an expert by profession (a psychiatrist, or a clinical psychologist). So, I already knew that this was the route I wanted to go down. Not long after my review I also found out that rehabilitation did use to be an aim of CMHT, but for some reason it no longer was.

I also took a test to see whether or not I was on the Autism spectrum, which proved negative. And regarding my medication, I was told that I could not be forced to take my medication, and if I didn't want to continue with my injection, they would just make a note on my record. However, I said that I did not wish to stop my injection unilaterally, and I would not bring it up again for a while. This was partly because I wanted them to oversee any withdrawal.

The problem of attachment, or lack of it, was never touched on, at the review, or after, but my research had led me to Dr Elaine Arnold, and her book Working with Families of African Caribbean Origin, which deals in depth with attachment, and how people of my generation, what is now called, the 'Windrush Generation', were affected by separation from their parents, and the lasting effect it had on many.

Dr Arnold has become a very good friend of mine, and we meet up regularly for lunch. She also follows my progress.

For my interview with the review board, I felt I did not want to antagonise them, or to be seen as questioning their authority so I pleaded with them for their help in order that I might resolve the issues that I had.

I am now a peer tutor at the Tower Hamlets Recovery College, and through teaching and working with some amazing professionals, I am now getting my life back, and have experienced healing.

8

THE PILLS THAT NEARLY KILLED ME - RECLAIMING MY LIFE – Anna Smith

Before that time, I never would have imagined that I would be talking or writing about the mental health services, or the damaging treatment I was about to receive.

First crisis: 'It all felt unspeakable'

In February 2005, I was assessed and treated by the Home Treatment Team during my initial crisis. I had become miserable, worried and anxious due to the isolation I was experiencing after completing my degree and being unemployed.

I so wanted to speak up about all the concerns that were running through my head, but I felt, for my own reasons, it was all unspeakable. I didn't have the words or confidence to make anything sound true to my thoughts. I know now that a lot of my issues stemmed from my identity. By identity, I mean that I am a mixed heritage/black woman. It is part of my makeup that has often left me feeling unsure of myself, confused and speechless.

I found it hard to reason out the way I was thinking and feeling. It was beginning to become more and more of an issue for me. It would have taken a lot more than what was being offered to get any of that information out of me at the time.

On reflection, I don't think I was asked any questions relevant to a young woman who had never been in contact with mental health services before. Discussions were rushed and it was frightening for me. Different team members visited all the time, so there was no sense of continuity or consistency. No relationship of trust was developed.

The response: Medications plus stereotypes

The team became very eager to give me medications but did not explain how they could affect me. The issue of adverse side effects was just never addressed.

Some team members also made assumptions about me: for example, one psychiatrist stated that I was a 'drama queen'. I got the impression that another member of the team thought I was another angry black woman with attitude. My mum later told me that the team assumed I didn't have any major problems because on the surface everything seemed fairly stable in my life: I'd finished university, had friendships and so on. Related to this, I was made to feel like a nuisance when I tried to report my suffering; the response was 'I've heard all about you,' when I phoned up their support line. All these assumptions only led to more anxiety and paranoia. Overall, their communication was not clear or compassionate. My voice was not heard.

Although I was comforted at first by the intervention, I was distressed by the severe side effects of the medication and the lack of interest and curiosity in me and my life. The treatment I was receiving drove me to believe that nobody understood my predicament. I waited expectantly for the antidepressant to make me feel better. But I experienced the opposite as the medication was making me feel worse: confused, anxious and more suicidal.

After two weeks, I was told I was psychotic and given antipsychotic medication. Then things got worse again. I felt like I had been shot in the head and my brain was disintegrating – I just wanted the old me back.

I began to think of various ways to end my life: I felt compelled to do something to stop the unbearable bodily sensations and hallucinations/thoughts I was having. This was combined with restlessness and no sleep since taking the medication. I thought that nobody knew what to do. The whole time I felt unable to express myself – partly because of the paranoia and partly because I didn't know any of these people. I don't think I had ever seen so many medical people in my life! It was terrifying and at one point I thought that they were terrorists! Their communication was horrendous.

'It didn't feel like 'normal' suicidal ideation'

After about 3-4 weeks of this treatment and home visits, I decided enough was enough. I remember the day – Friday 4th March 2005. It was exactly a week before my 24th birthday. It had been torturous. I couldn't sleep but I couldn't stay awake. I thought I was in heaven, but I didn't belong there. I had tried to escape on a couple of occasions so I could jump off the nearest high building (sometimes I thought I already had). Anyway, that morning of 4th March 2005, I found the means and courage to hang myself. Suicide became the only way out for me – to resolve the issue.

In fact, I really couldn't stop myself. It didn't feel like 'normal' suicidal ideation – this felt like I was contaminated by a drug that was driving me to do it. I didn't feel depressed, but more like a zombie, uncontrollably taking direction from a parasite inside my body. I never imagined that would happen as a result of taking medications.

Reflection: A chemical imbalance or social power imbalance?

When I look back now, I often feel like my experience was a very strong example of negligence in the sense that the mental health professionals neglected or ignored my whole life experience forming my identity. The poster I created entitled 'Chemical Imbalance or Social Power Imbalance' reflects this for me: how aspects of my life such as my ethnicity, my age, my recent university experience, unemployment, family issues, my peer group, religion and spirituality and more were not explored but swept under the carpet.

I had wholeheartedly trusted the common belief that I had a chemical imbalance that could be treated with medication. But I only became more disempowered by the treatment. Hopelessness and apathy set in – my quality of life decreased and my sense of self diminished.

Thankfully I survived my suicide attempt without any lasting physical damage. Yet, I still feel that for many years my reaction to the medication was also swept under the carpet – with no acknowledgement that the medication had a major influence on my suicide attempt.

Instead, I was treated with more medication and given another diagnosis. I feel that I was silenced. I did my best to try to forget about the traumatic event and its impact, hoping that I would make a full recovery and it would all go away.

Unfortunately, however I faced a lack of compassion plus ongoing stigmatisation: This included being seen as a very sick/unwell person and treated in a patronising manner. Feeling undermined by all the negative media surrounding mental health – newspapers, news reports, films linking violence and murder to mental illness – I became much more vulnerable to deeper distress. Ultimately, these experiences hindered my recovery journey in unimaginable ways.

Life after hospitalisation

I had never been admitted to a psychiatric hospital before my initial crisis and suicide attempt. However, I was admitted from the ITU directly into a mental health ward and medicated again. It was impossible for me not to react to what happened in one way or another. At first, I was depressed and obsessed with a pressure mark on my neck. Then as I realised I had somehow 'cheated death' unscathed, I found a new energy. Suddenly, I wanted to work hard and play hard. I wanted to live a completely hedonistic lifestyle. Through meeting other patients and all being medicated 'up to the eyeballs', I discovered new habits and new ways of living – smoking and eating too much and a more carefree attitude.

After being discharged from hospital the first time, seeking work became increasingly difficult. The situation only worsened with subsequent hospitalisations: I faced gaps in my employment, a lack of confidence and generally feeling quite sedated from the medications. This led to 'play' becoming the more predominant feature in my life. I was eating too much, smoking too much, binge drinking and dabbling in illegal drugs.

My housing was also becoming more of an ongoing and complicated problem. From my first encounter with the mental health services in 2005 until 2008, I lived in London.

Then in January 2008, I relocated with my mother to a seaside town. We had hoped for a new start, fresh air, light and a better quality of life. It was a mutual decision between us that I needed to find more independent living arrangements. Mum wrote a letter appealing to the council. After some time, in September 2009, I was offered hostel accommodation and was also on the social housing waiting list. I was made false promises by the hostel worker and told that this route would lead me to more permanent housing. It did not.

The hostel was filled with people with lots of problems and needs, all of whom needed to be housed. I came across many predatory people in the year I spent at the hostel, and it was hard not to get socially involved with some of the residents. It became too frightening and destabilising for me in the end – I was around people who were exposing more and more volatile sides of themselves. I was unable to sort my own life out due to the distraction of it all. I was being led down the wrong path and blowing caution to the wind. I didn't have the headspace to allow myself to take stock of the situation and make a change. There was too much temptation to bury my head in the sand and allow the wild times to carry on, even though I didn't want them to. It was really impacting on my mental health though.

'All the trauma could no longer be contained'

Mum came to the rescue again: at the beginning of 2011, she helped me find a place in supported housing for people with a mental health diagnosis. It was calmer to start with but terribly lonely in a very small studio room at the back of a house. I then got involved in a relationship with one of the residents in the building.
Relatively quickly I found out about his past and his 'red flags' as a partner. This was the last straw for me. It pushed me right into the path of a full-blown crisis and I ended up being sectioned for the first time in October 2011.

All the trauma I was trying to keep a lid on could no longer be contained. The first trauma had been the major incident of my suicide attempt. Then because of that attempt and being unable to find any understanding of that incident, I think I acted out. This led to more trauma caused by over-drinking alcohol, taking illegal street drugs and the risky and reckless behaviour that can happen as result of all of that.

Then there was the running theme of my insecure housing situation weighing down on me. I was well outside of my boundaries and well out of my comfort zone.

I was sectioned in 2011 and, in 2012, it happened again. From 2012 up until 2020, I was hospitalised every two years. The hospital admissions added more traumas to the mix. I was put in isolation for the first time in 2012; it was horrendous and disturbing – I felt like I went to the corners of my mind. I was transferred to a more intensive care ward in a hospital further away because of my 'disturbing' behaviour. In the intensive care ward, I felt I was going more out of my mind due to the boredom and side effects of the medication, which again, nobody paid attention to. I also became mildly aggressive because of the side effects of the medication and lack of interaction/stimulation plus being followed around by some strange man who took pleasure in telling me frightening stories. Again, I was put in seclusion. I don't jest when I say it is a horrific experience.

Impact on my identity

A couple of times, I think in 2014 and 2016, I tried to reduce my medication in the hope of withdrawing completely from it. I had the most difficult time reducing and began not sleeping, having discomfort in my body and vivid visual hallucinations. This again was terrifying each time and contributed to me entering a psychotic state – I was not at all in the common reality. Once, I went running and dancing down the seafront – I had lost all inhibitions and felt that I had found a higher level of understanding. It felt so exhilaratingly liberating at the time.

Yet, every time I was sectioned, in hospital and finally out again – once the novelty of being discharged and starting over had worn off, the depression set in. Trauma responses reappeared: panic attacks, anxiety, reticence, shame, embarrassment, withdrawal. This seemed to happen every time after the 2011 admission – there would be a drama/action-packed experience followed by the mess that I then had to process.

The care coordinators that were allocated to me seemed to send me round in circles. They sent me to the same groups and wrote recovery action plans. They also subtly restricted me by making me feel incapable and dangerous through questionable expressions and statements until I just became increasingly depressed and felt hopeless. The psychiatrists then just offered more medications.

Often they only saw me every 6 months for about 10 minutes each time. The emphasis was on the *problem being inside of me*. I remember one psychiatrist arguing in 2009 that I could be 'dangerous' if I didn't take extra medication.

That really didn't help my state of mind and probably added to my lack of confidence and anxiety. No matter how much I didn't believe what he had said, it stuck with me and caused me to feel very self-conscious to the point of irrationality. None of this was ever mentioned. Nor was my suicide attempt due to the reaction to psychiatric medication and the trauma it caused. I completely lost a sense of my already fragile identity. My identity had become that of the compliant, fearful, silent, submissive patient.

Reclaiming my life

Although I was a compliant patient in many respects, I had attempted to withdraw from my medications on a few occasions using different methods. The antidepressant was the one that I came off suddenly, after forgetting to take it for a few days. I felt it wasn't helping my depression and that I wanted to get out of it naturally, by myself – to find other tools to help me. I think it was in 2014 that I first attempted to withdraw from the antipsychotic I was taking. Unfortunately, this withdrawal contributed to another hospital admission. I think I was given the wrong information about how to withdraw but a large part of me was still preoccupied with all the trauma, and I couldn't focus on the task of learning about the process or looking after myself. The same thing happened in 2016. In 2018, I used a different approach, but reduced too quickly. It was all similar in 2020.

About two years ago, I learned from a psychiatrist that when I was administered the medication in 2005, I suffered an iatrogenic effect that led to akathisia. 'Iatrogenic' means that I had an adverse reaction caused by medical treatment.

'Akathisia' is an internal agitation/restlessness known to be caused by some medications. It can be totally unbearable and lead to suicide. This information, along with my ongoing desire to get back to a feeling of me, spurred me on to want to withdraw from my medications. I wanted to have an experience of what life was like without my medication. I was also worried about the long-term effects it was having on my health – one of the worries was the enormous amount of weight I had gained and the possibility of developing heart problems or diabetes. Research has also discovered other health problems such as tardive dyskinesia, brain shrinkage and a shorter life span by 20-25 years. I needed to feel the strength that the uncertainty would give to me – to take a chance on something in order to feel that a 'medication-free' life was possible. Even though it was also terrifying because of the normality of taking a pill every day for me, it felt worth the risk. In 2016, I engaged with a new initiative (Dialogue First – Open Dialogue Approach), and I had also been seeing a private therapist since 2010. Being able to be open about my experiences and my hopes and fears was helpful in gaining confidence and getting to know myself.

In May 2020, after being hospitalised from February until mid-March of that year, I decided that I would try to withdraw from the antipsychotic again. I had encouragement from the Dialogue First team and my mother with whom I was then residing, so it seemed that I could have a good chance of succeeding this time. I felt I could learn from experience and take measures to really look after myself. In fact, the lockdown was helpful for me.

As soon as I was discharged from hospital, the lockdown began, and everything had to slow down. It was like going into convalescence – I was being eased back into the community and not experiencing the usual fast pace of life familiar to me when I am discharged from hospital.

Even getting on the bus was easier – less panic-making, as the buses were nearly empty, and everyone was wearing masks. The masks really suited my social anxiety – especially with hats in the winter.

Fast forward to July 2022, and I am on the lowest dose of antipsychotic I have ever been on. I had a few weeks of sleeping badly but feel a lot better now. My panic attacks have greatly improved and don't cause as much disruption to my life. The lockdown, along with other support I have in place, has given me a chance to really care for myself whilst going through this process, surprisingly!

Coming to terms with the harm

When I reflect on the treatment I received over the years, it is a bitter pill to swallow. When I am depressed, my life doesn't really matter to me, but when I am not depressed, I start to feel angry about what happened to me. I think about all the years that have gone by with me mostly blaming myself. I think about how the treatment I received obscured the power imbalances that I was noticing.

Chunks of my development felt arrested and it's painful for me to realise that it has taken me so long to grasp an understanding of my own. I have needed to understand the role of life events and how racial inequalities, gender inequalities, wealth disparities, education/knowledge inequalities, religion/spirituality biases exist and come in different forms. It has been difficult to come to terms with this and discover it is an ongoing problem for all of us. I can't second-guess anything really; situations and beliefs are constantly changing. What I am surer of now is that a pill won't make it go away!

I really thought that I would be offered a valuable service and that the pills would mend the situation. Looking back, I would have appreciated more honesty, even if it wasn't what I wanted to hear. Somehow, I needed to be told that life is difficult and that there is no quick fix – I really needed to hear that! I have concluded that making assumptions and over-medicating people is giving false hope and potentially ruining lives – one size doesn't fit all, we are all different. It's difficult to accept that there is nothing much beyond the current mental health services. Moreover, the mainstream culture has been extremely difficult to re-engage with. For me, the mental health system is not working. Sometimes I question whether a mental health service even exists because it has been so disappointing for me.

Ironically, there has been some good to come out of this whole messy situation. I have had more of a chance to give time to finding out about myself and working on my wellbeing. It is kind of perversely a blessing in disguise.

Had things not become life-threatening at the very start, I am not sure how long it would have taken for me to wake up to the inefficiency of the mental health services. Even so, it still took a long time to reach a point of clarity over what happened – and this was mainly because a lot of people didn't want to address it. Luckily, I had a supportive mum who believed me and would not let it drop. Yet, ultimately, I had to reach an understanding of my own. I think I am almost there, even though that isn't necessarily a permanent state of mind. I am more open to the uncertainty of life and human emotions.

I am really in awe of the fact that my life could have been very different (I mean much, much worse) had it not been for a certain amount of luck on my side.

For example, I could have hung myself at night or while my mum was out. I shudder at the thought of this sometimes. I was crying out for help but was forced to act in a very drastic way. Somehow, I had a little bit of life force remaining in me to make my mum aware and alert to my pain. I also had a certain something that stopped me from ever 'going too far' outside of my moral beliefs and values. I was always held back somehow from actions and behaviour that could have been life-changing during my psychotic episodes. What still angers me is that many mental health service staff never really address the underlying issues facing a person - or how mental health can be destabilised significantly by the impact of challenging life experiences. I think my journey through mental health services is a clear example of this.

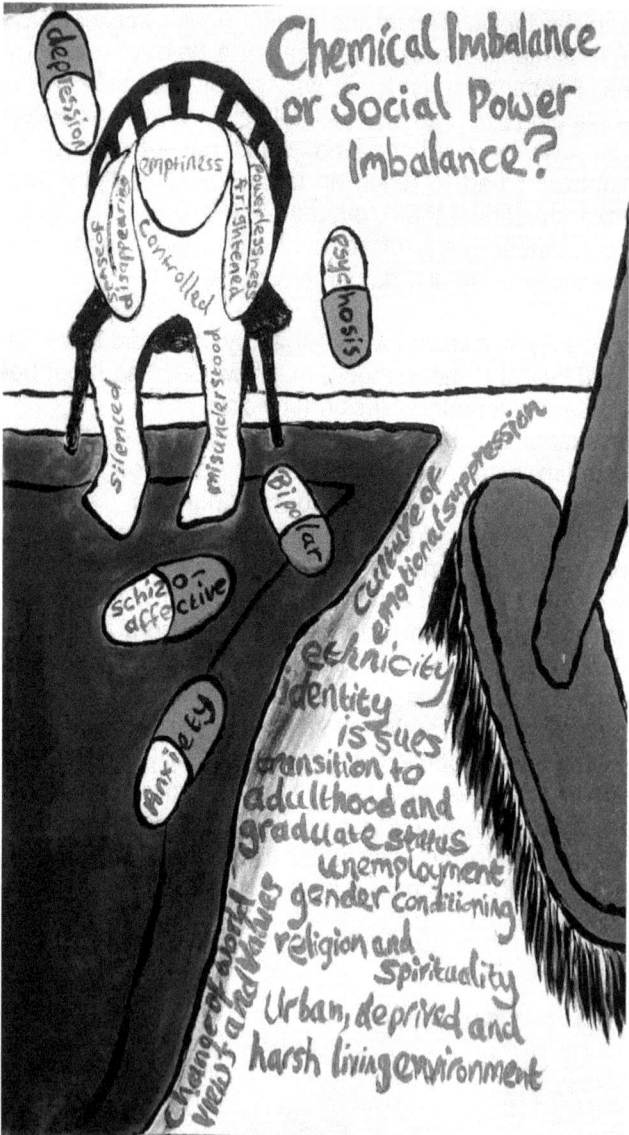

© Anna Smith

9

MENTAL FAIRYTALE – Jacq A

I won't tell a soul

Trigger Warnings: Mentions of suicide ideation, ableism, biphobia, fatphobia, racism, childhood and adult sexual abuse.

The next time I'm suicidal (and there will always be a next time), I will know to keep my trap shut.

The last time I asked for help (the final time, Jacq), I was met with the combined forces of the NHS East London Mental Health Trust. And who could stand against such a mighty ogre? Not I, that's for damn sure. My terrible experiences with them sealed my fate, the way a princess would be sealed away in a castle. I would never ask for help again.

I browse through Instagram during Mental Health Awareness week. It reads like a fairytale complete with a 'Happily ever after'. There are Posts and Reels and Stories urging me to 'just reach out!' Depression is the only condition mentioned. I chuckle darkly as I remember folding a piece of paper into eight squares so I could create a mini-zine about Dissociative Identity Disorder for the staff on the ward I'd been placed on because none of them had ever heard of it before. (What good did it do, Jacq?)

I realise I am a mythical creature in the eyes of mental health professionals. Black people aren't supposed to have Post-traumatic Stress Disorder, Binge Eating Disorder or any of the other conditions I have. The line of suited medical students gasps when I recount what I have survived and all the scars, both internal and external, it has left me with. Surely sexual abuse doesn't happen to Black kids? Once I turned eighteen, it must have stopped, right? (Nah, Jacq. It just got covered with a cloak of invisibility.) I must be a liar - an untrustworthy changeling who will say anything to get what they want!

'You're no better than a lying prostitute. No Christian man will want you now,' my dad told me right before I ran away.

The last psych ward (please let it be the final one, Jacq) had thirteen rooms. I was placed in the unluckiest one at the end of the corridor. I was assaulted twice by other patients during the six days I was there. I was an easy target with multiple bullseyes painted on my back (Oh, Jacq, why can't you be less Black, fat, bald and queer?) I was the creature others would destroy while they were playing the lowest setting of the game - the warm-up before the real quest took hold. None of the staff cared enough to believe me, let alone ask if my injuries needed treatment.

From the present, I proclaim that in my fairytale of existing as a mentally ill person, the professionals with their suits and clipboards were the real demons of the piece. The most senior staff member on the ward spent our entire interview with her back turned to me while she typed into her computer. I wonder now if we'd ever made eye contact, would she have burst into flames? Would I have turned into stone? Either way, it did me no good.

Sometimes I feel like the Fool in the Tarot deck, blissfully setting out on a journey when they don't know anything about the dangers. 'Just reach out!' has led to me being lied to over and over again. It has led to a white gay staff member promising to check in on me on the ward only to vanish once he went back to his office, never to be seen again. It has led to a white clinical psychologist telling me, 'I know all about racism because I get discriminated against due to my Swiss accent.' Reaching out has resulted in my having to banish a visitor from the Home Treatment team because she told me the racism I experienced, which made my mental health worse, wasn't really racism and she knew this because she had studied the subject at university. Asking for help has resulted in the only Black therapist I've ever seen telling me that there was no such thing as bisexuality and I should admit that I was too scared to be a lesbian.

When I ran away from my violent and abusive family thirty years ago, I had no choice. I thought things would be better if I completed my quest. I saw myself as the hero of the fairytale and believed I would rescue myself from that dastardly tower I'd been locked away in. But I was wrong. There is no happy ever after for someone like me. My character in the story is too strange a mix for readers to bear. I am portrayed as the victim and the villain and the dragon to be vanquished. I am also the witch who tricks and grabs at them like thorns in the bushes along the path. And reaching out doesn't help when mental health 'professionals' cannot stand to be in the same room as the monster I am presented as.

There is no tidy end to my story. Next year there will be another Mental Health Awareness week. The NHS will prescribe sharing a cup of tea with neighbours who would run a mile if they knew the mental health conditions I live with. They will recommend going for a walk in a world where white gay men have spat on me at a Pride march and where people would rather stand for hours on a busy train than sit beside a fat, Black person like me. And nobody will care to understand the moral of the tale.

Ends.

Image description: a blue square on a light-brown door as background. The words on the blue square read 'Bedroom 13'. This is where I stayed while on the Orchid Ward in Newham Mental Health hospital in 2020

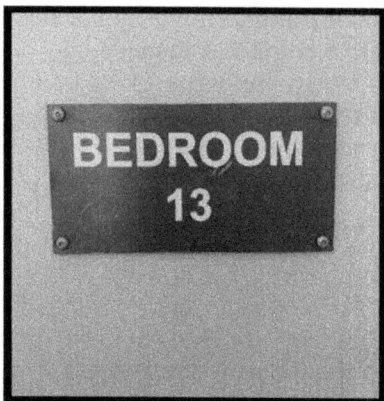

10

BEING YOURSELF OFTEN MEANS JUST NOT BEING YOUR STEREOTYPE: A JEWISH DYSLEXIC RANT - Michelle Baharier

I believe I have always been 'nuts, mad, looney' or whatever name you care to give me. I'll recycle myself in the looney-bin breaking the stigma and hate thrown at me.

So, I am going to explorer how a dyslexic working-class Jewish kid was doomed to need mental health services. Yes – the system, predicts this, how do I know?

In 1998 I acquired my medical notes, it was a depressing and shocking read. These doctors had mapped out a life, my life, as one of mental ill health. They decided I was a somatiser, that at nine I would be condemned, by depression, part of this, if not all, was based on the fact I had been diagnosed with dyslexia as, of course, tragically many dyslexic children make attempts on their lives. My diagnoses were made when I was age nine, in 1972, seems from then on, I was medically dammed.

So, the health and school system assigned me a range of labels - I was kaput for life. The labels were dyslexia, depression, anxiety, audio deficit, anger, rage and disruption; but the othering and bullying in schools played a really significant role in that. At primary school, I experienced Catholic kids in my school throwing stones at me when I was riding my bike; they had already decided, I killed Jesus some 2000 years ago. The police were called, but my parents were told because no blood was spilled, they would not do anything.

I was a kid, I had no clue, the world was something I was discovering. I was seen by a school psychologist who had no eyebrows, because the fashion of the time was to shave them off. I remember this because she gave me a card and I had to say to her what was missing on this picture of the face. And it was eyebrows. I was scared to say as she didn't have any, not real ones anyway. She was a hippy looking woman with a long skirt, dyed blonde hair, and she scared me. She gave me all these tests; I couldn't do or even understand half of them. The outcome of this meeting was I was tied to this woman for any support during my school education and she would give the label **dyslexia**. This was momentous for me – partly because it opened the door for support, but it also opened the door for stigma and prejudice. For me this meant I was taken out of class to attend a **'special needs'**[15] classes with other **'thick'** and **'disruptive'** kids as we were perceived, but certainly not how I felt. My parents were also informed that I should no longer learn Hebrew as it was affecting my ability to learn English!

Not only did I come from a family of immigrants, like many Jews, my family where working-class and they left school at 14 with a very limited formal education. This meant my family/parents did not really question the school psychologist nor any doctor, as they were seen as a highly educated person and a pillar of that community. Nor were they encouraged or equipped to question the doctors' decisions.

By the time I was 14 I was a mental health patient (these days I'd call myself a participant in my care but back then I didn't know that was an option).

I was labelled with clinical depression, suicidal thoughts, and was put on diazepam - meaning I slept a lot and gained weight. As a teenager this was the last thing I

---

[15] I use these terms as they were the language I grew up with, not because I agree with it

wanted. It made going out to parties difficult. I often passed out and had to be bought home by others – these occurrences were very unnerving as I had no memory of what happened. In fact, I was quite out of control at this point.

From then on, every physical symptom I presented to a doctor was treated as a mental health issue – this was called somatising or somatisation. For me this meant I received no check-ups or investigations despite presenting with symptoms of rheumatic fever[16]. It had taken a good twelve months to convince them this was a physical condition and not the effects of my mental health.

At the same time, I was dealing with puberty, antisemitism and ignorance, and sexual harassment from boys my age. This often took the form of me and my body being seen as some 'exotic' object – in some fetishised way. The worst was being asked if I was circumcised, this made me so incredibly angry, but I was too young to break down why. It was such an invasive, overtly sexual question.

All of this on top of dealing with mental health services, of which there was no support or understanding, let alone having a say in my 'care,' left me quite devoid of being able to cope with my mental health, particularly as I did not understand it.

I believe that my emotional turmoil was a normal reaction to my actual life. My Uncle took his own life and my father was dying of brain cancer. I was having to deal with all the of this whilst my Mum, who tried her best, was falling apart. She was prescribed a Valium style drug and pain killers. I was an adolescent in an extremally dysfunctional family.

---

[16] A rare complication that can develop after a bacterial throat infection; symptoms include painful joints and heart problems

A bit of Cultural Context

I have a dysfunctional ultra-orthodox/laxed-orthodox, conventional (conservative), traditional religious practicing Ashkenazi Father and a Sephardic Mother to add to the blend of this complex web, which makes up my intersectional identity. I learned later in life that my father had lived with manic depression – I was told he had electro-convulsive therapy. I believe now that what he probably had was transferred from his family. His father was from Poland, but he was a Russian citizen as were so many people at that time given the borders with Russia were always moving. His family mostly died through Russian Programs and then the Holocaust. His Mother was German, sadly we know what happened to most of them, but I don't know what happened to her relatives.

At the time my father was using mental health services, the idea of his parents passing down their trauma would not have been widely known. Therefore, his treatment would not have reflected his cultural identity. I assume he had a very heavy burden of death and feelings of guilt around being alive which is relatively common for anyone who survives a conflict. For me, understanding transference and my experience growing up in the UK has helped me understand my mental health.

Although I am UK born, I have always felt foreign. My Grandfather lived with us, his accent was not English; people were always asking if I was Australian or French, right from when I was a little kid. As an adult, I am more careful about where I disclose my heritage because Antisemitism has become worse, or perhaps I notice it more. Within mental health services, they hold a stereotype of what a Jew is; you are tossed around as a pet or a toy by staff members, particularly fundamentalist Christians who at one point informed me that I needed to be kept alive for the Resurrection of Christ. I felt like they only saw me as an object - very few looked at me as an individual.

It is hard to feel safe enough in psychiatry to express your Jewishness. Jewish culture is inherently argumentative and complex – often there are five opinions and only two people in the room! This often does not translate into British culture which likes black/white, well-defined parameters such as Good or Bad Jews depending on your stance on Israel.

This overly simple way of looking at things feeds into staff attitudes. The first psychiatrist I had, it felt like she was imposing her own Catholic identity on me. She did not know anything about my culture or understand any of the idiosyncrasies. So, when I asked lots of questions, it felt like she took offense – when asking lots of questions is natural in Jewish culture.

I have experienced a range of conscious and unconscious bias from other service users and staff which make accessing help more stressful and often harder. Some people project their political opinion onto me and my Jewishness, so as a consequence it can feel like a whole society is ganging up on me.

Access to (good) Food

Whenever I have been an inpatient the staff lacked an understanding of Jewish culture, particularly in relation to food. While they offer Kosha food as an option, in my experience it is never actually available therefore I ended up eating the 'Asia vegetarian' option due to my allergies. How is this not discrimination?

Jewish people's friends and families end up bringing us food as it is never provided by the NHS. Our need for Kosha food is trivialised and ignored – I have been given excuses like 'oh we don't do that in South London, only in the North.'

The fact that Jewish people's food needs are not acknowledged, let alone provided for, shows just how insignificant we are regarded as a group of people with individual cultural needs. Food is a number one priority when you are making sure that someone is in a safe environment – as it shows you are caring for their mental and physical health.

The fact that our food needs are not adhered to has always made me feel quite angry; there is so much gaslighting. They say they are providing for us with Kosha food when, in reality, we do not receive it. I don't know if this is different in other cultures dietary needs, but I hope they are provided for.

I have spent my time in mental health services defending myself whilst educating staff. I often do not speak out in fear of the antisemitic backlash. It also adds insult to injury that the stereotypes portrayed about Jews is that: we killed Jesus, we live in the Promised land, and we were murdered by Nazis.

There is no recognition of Jewish cultural diversity – we are not all Eastern European. There is a total void in people's knowledge of Jews and Judaism, and this is also reflected in mental health services.

Obviously in therapy and therapeutic situations you need to feel safe. I was undergoing my third breakdown and being seen by several therapists. Some who made me experience being unacceptable, due to my Jewish heritage. I, as a Jew, am a person of the book. I was bought up celebrating Pesach (Passover), celebrating that we escaped Egypt, that we are not slaves, we are free people. I am a free person. Most of my immediate family either live in Israel or are Orthodox or Frum; I would consider myself secular.

My father's family kept their family tree – written in Aramaic, Hebrew, and Yiddish. It tells us that they lived in Jerusalem thousands of years ago before being expelled by the Romans – who created the blood libel[17]. As a people, we have experience persecution after persecution, it is no wonder as a culture we struggle to feel safe in any environment – whether country wide or in small communities like in the borough of London I lived in.

How am I supposed to feel safe using mental health services?

I know I have an inner fear of the system, including the staff, which makes me feel unsafe; because of my experiences of racism, I have become very guarded and it's hard to give away my trust.

This really shows how the system doesn't allow Jewish people to enter safe treatment, that enables us to explore the diversity of our culture. You do not want to disclose or discuss your Jewishness, because you often end up being shut down. Because of the hierarchy mental health sits in, I have learned to oppress my Jewishness. I find it is also suppressed, ignored, and made obsolete by the system who cannot respond in a non-judgemental way. You don't want to be treated by someone who shames the core of your person.

Staff members projecting their opinions on Jewishness under the guise of a conversation, but in reality, dominating you with their opinion on Israeli politics makes

---

[17] An antisemitic canard which falsely accurses Jews of murdering Christian boys with the goal of using their blood in the performance of religious rituals

me feel guarded and distrustful. The staff are often making Anti-Semitic accusations about my identity – using excuses like 'my colleague is Jewish' to justify their actions. But to me they are being an antisemite while hiding behind Anti-Zionism/Israelis. They shouldn't be airing their opinions, regardless, but in doing so they are creating a hazardous environment, making it harder to bring things up and engage in 'treatment.'

Sadly, some mental health practitioners appear to have little knowledge of Jewish history prior to the 1970s. They may even buy into the blood libel. They certainly know nothing of Russian involvement in the Yom Kippur war – which was started on the 'High Holiday' in 1973. So, you are in a room with the Doctor – your psychiatrist, who does not know or care for your culture, and is not willing to hear about it from you. They will decide if you are a good Jew who hates Israel or a bad Jew who supports Israel based on their opinion. This was my experience! But I am there to explore and be supported including my experiences of antisemitism; but I am doing it with a judgmental person who has already decided their opinion me, put me in boxes based on their prejudices and then observed me and made their decisions without my input.

A different psychiatrist who assumed I had a lot of feelings of guilt and requested I explain them without any more context. Guilt over what? My Jewish guilt? I am guilty as I am Jewish? She was Catholic and it seemed to me she was imposing her ideas about guilt, sex, and purity. Perhaps she meant 'it is the guilt of survival that weighs heavily' No, you must be joking. Jews get married, we have sex, we don't relate sex and sin in the way Christianity does. Did she think I killed Jesus? For fucks sake I was not alive when Jesus died. I wanted to change psychiatrist, but this was the 1980s, there was no support or information on how to. She refused to let me be transferred suggesting all other psychiatrists would be the same implying there would be no benefit in me doing it. Even as recently 2015, my disability – my dyslexia – has not been considered. I met another psychiatrist who caused me a lot of distressed and anxiety. He used acronyms to assesses my mental health without considering the fact that I didn't understand them. That translating them into words is a cognitive process I cannot do due to my disability – never mind the amount of the mental distress and suicidal feelings I was having at the time. He gave me the 'Clinical depression' note and heavy-duty drugs and sleeping pills, with contact from a home treatment team.

I had grown up and am living in a society which would not protect me if I was harmed. As a child this was traumatic and contributed to me needing mental health support. As an adult I have had to learn to be resilient to it. Ending up in mental health services and their inability to provide a culturally sensitive service through their lack of support, for me, increased my desire to choose to end it.

Feeling safe outside of mental health services

To protect myself I have had to rely on Jewish care for culturally sensitive support. In 2015 I was severely unwell and had lost of a lot of non-Jewish friends due to the frenzy surrounding Jeremy Corbyn. I acknowledge that Jeremy Corbyn was slandered severely by the media – look at the racism Boris Johnson has gotten away with after all. But both left and right media have ran campaigns demonising Israel and ignoring the nuances of the situation which have incited violence against Jewish people.

To me, the Jeremy Corbyn frenzy gave license for people to air their antisemitic views and I have experienced an increase in antisemitism since then. This has led to me being gaslight about what counts and what does not as antisemitic treatment. It's made me feel that more people are perceiving me as right wing when I feel politically homeless. It felt like my allies were prepared to throw me, as a Jew, under the bus for policies which would benefit them. As a young person I experienced self-hate and I feel for the young Jewish people who are swallowing themselves and their identity because identifying as Jewish has increased in risk off the back of what started with Jeremy Corbyn but is continuing to this day.

Many people who use mental health services already have low self-esteem, self-loathing, and often neglect themselves. Some feel shame to the core. When this – the shame - is impacted by an unspoken silence you feel like you can't speak freely about the gaslighting you are experiencing as a Jew, so you end up being subjected to further racist abuse. Just consider, as a British citizen you were told that the prejudice you experienced was not real, that 3000 years plus of history was fake.

There are so many examples of antisemitism across the world. My Mum, as mentioned before, was Sephardic, her family came from Spain, Portugal, and Holland - so why are they in the UK? They are here because of the inquisition - another genocide against Jews. Even in the 1200's the Jews were killed and kicked out of the UK. There is no country we have not been killed for being Jewish – of course we feel homeless. It is not surprising, then, that many Jewish people are neurotic and 'dysfunctional', certainly in my circle we all have quite a nervous disposition. I have several labels plus I fear being bad, unworthy, and acting hateful towards myself. I find myself getting eaten up and internalising these non-stop negative messages – not surprising after years of hate against people like me and my personal experiences of hate.

The Survivor Movement and me

I really struggled and still do struggle with the language of survivors of psychiatry. I know I hold some of my oppression but survivors to me have always been those who have come out of concentration camps. I didn't feel that I had the right to that label, as 'survivor' for me is a very precious, even though I do understand everyone is a survivor, in my culture is holds a specific, protected meaning.

I have been part of the user voice movement since the mid 1980's and hung out at the Diorama and other disabled people's spaces. I also founded CoolTan Arts; a participant led arts and mental health organisation. We wanted to give people an artistic space to express themselves, including running workshops, having exhibits, and selling pieces. We wanted to create art opportunities. We won 27 awards including the GSK IMPACT Award. These days I am getting on with my own arts practice and look forward to seeing you at my exhibitions.

STORIES OF EXISTING IN A RACIALISED BODY

11

'ARE YOU SURE IT'S NOT JUST ANXIETY?': MY DIFFICULT JOURNEY TO ADHD/AUTISM DIAGNOSIS AS A RACIALISED QUEER WOMXN – Priscilla Eyles

I probably shouldn't be alive.

Medical racism left me literally fighting for breath at birth, leaving an imprint of trauma which undoubtedly, irreversibly scarred my body-mind. The body-mind of a queer neurodivergent bi-racial queer womxn with autism, ADHD, anxiety and most probably C/PTSD given all the sh*t I've been through.

My story partly the result of being part of this long colourful spectrum of varied, maladaptive, intergenerational, racialised and environmental trauma responses.

My parents come from harsh backgrounds filled with discrimination and hardship. My mother, a Black Zimbabwean Ndebele refugee, came to England in the late 70s, fleeing from Mugabe's genocidal militia to work as a nurse.

My dad is white British and neurodivergent, growing up at a time when dyslexia was often seen as a sign of stupidity, resulting in traumatising school punishments.

Now let's begin at the beginning.

My first encounter with medical racism

My birth day.

My mother knew I was going to be a breech baby from her maternity nurse training. When she told the head obstetrician this and insisted they book in a caesarean section, he dismissed her, saying that because she was African and 'shaped like a barrel' she would be able to push me out 'without a problem'.

This attitude has its origin in colonial 18th-century logic, when slave owners justified the violent treatment of African slaves, by claiming that they had a naturally higher tolerance to pain. (A belief that sadly continues to negatively affect the medical care of racialised people today).

Because of this racist logic, I nearly died from umbilical strangulation. It's only because my mother understood the dangers, and demanded attending staff to perform an emergency caesarean, that I survived.

Consequently, I was deprived of oxygen and had to spend a week isolated in ICU, unable to immediately bond with my mother, was significant to my developmental issues[18]. That first contact is said to be vital for establishing secure attachment and developmental health.

So, this episode has undoubtably played a long-term role in my anxious-ambivalent attachment style[19], leaving me with severe anxiety and a sense of helplessness and abandonment when forced to be alone for too long.

---

[18]   https://www.birthinjuryguide.org/2014/05/birth-injuries-developmental-delays/#:~:text=Study%20Reveals%20Birth%20Injuries%20as%20Most%20Common%20Cause,Autism.%20%E2%80%9CReduced%20oxygen%20supply%2C%20during%20labor%2C%20during%20delivery%2C

[19]   https://cptsdfoundation.org/2018/10/22/anxious-ambivalent-attachment-style-an-examination-of-its-causes-and-how-it-affects-adult-relationships/

Intergenerational trauma

My mother grew up in colonised Rhodesia, spending her formative years shaped by her experiences of being a 'second-class citizen'. She recalls being spat on by white Rhodesians and called a 'keffir'.

I believe she must've experienced attachment trauma, having been separated from her parents as a baby to go live with her grandmother, her parents too busy working and providing for her and her two brothers. As previously mentioned, she then had to escape Mugabe's regime in her 20s.

This all, I believe, contributed to my mother being unable to tolerate my depressive lows and anxiety growing up. As Kinouani highlights, immigrants escaping persecution can lack the 'emotional capacity to cope with additional trauma'.[20]

Additionally, both my parents lacked the understanding to get me the right medical help, which would have been difficult to get anyway. Near impossible growing up in the late 80s and early 90s, when ADHD wasn't even recognised as a diagnosis by NICE until 2000.[21]

From childhood to my twenties, I was left wondering what the hell was 'wrong' with me, as I kept repeating supposedly 'basic' mistakes and getting easily overwhelmed. I concluded that I must be fundamentally flawed - a perpetual liability.

---

[20] *Living While Black*, Guilaine Kinouani (Ebury Digital, 2021), p.99

I felt doomed to 'failure', my teenage diaries dark holes of despair and full of the most vitriolic self-directed abuse. I didn't realise I was let down by the safety nets, systems and people around me that were meant to catch me.

Racialised trauma

Despite the massive impact of racialised/intergenerational trauma on mental health and brain development, Western psychiatric treatment still largely fails to acknowledge how centuries of white supremacist attitudes impact those within marginalised communities.

Racist colonial attitudes can be further seen in the overrepresentation in psychiatric holds of racialised people, termed 'dangerously psychotic' or 'violent' etc. As well as in the underdiagnosis of neurodivergent conditions for people like me.

Medical practitioners willing/able to encourage conversations about racism are rare, and in the NHS are limited by the system they find themselves in. I still remember years ago, how excited and happy one of my late friends - Nila, was when they found a GP who understood and could openly acknowledge that their fibromyalgia was a result of racialised trauma.

With so many locums and 10-minute appointments, it is hard to build a trusting relationship that enables exploration of these issues. I myself have never felt comfortable broaching racism with my NHS psychiatrist, despite being vocally anti-racist and an intersectional neurodivergent activist.

Self-preservation kicks in: If I did say something, would it be taken seriously? Or would I just be dismissed as another oversensitive 'angry Black woman' playing the 'race card'.

Failure to acknowledge the impact of racism is what psychologist Guilaine Kinouani calls a feeling of 'epistemic homelessness'[22]. It describes how racialised people can feel disconnected from our internal guidance systems due to the overwhelming denial and silencing of our experiences (at its extreme it can lead to dissociating and psychosis).

A painfully destructive feeling I know too well, translating to long periods of self-doubt and circular rumination about my perceptions of discrimination.

Navigating the education and work industrial complex

A few incidents stick out from my time at school which would've made me a prime candidate for an ADHD and ASD diagnosis, if they had been better understood as something that doesn't just affect white boys and seen as co-occurring conditions.

About Age 7, I got so excited at the babysitters, preferring the company of adults to my peers as a child and prone to reckless impulsivity, that I decided to take my knickers off, as you do…

The next day a social worker came to take me out of my class and told me to draw a picture of my family (to determine any familial abuse) and then nothing happened…no follow up, despite my obvious need for support to manage behaviour which could and would later endanger me.

In secondary school, my illegible handwriting was such a constant cause of frustration that instead of curiosity or

---

[22]

https://www.ted.com/talks/guilaine_kinouani_epistemic_homeless ness support, it prompted a humiliating public telling off from one of my history teachers in front of all the whole history department. I only later found out that dysgraphia/fine motor issues are a common issue for neurodivergent people.

Teachers were also puzzled by why I had so much talent in the arts and humanities but found maths and science mostly incomprehensible - a classic neurodivergent 'spiky profile'.

I went from my Journalism MA only to have a string of unpaid media internships, where I was often bullied or reprimanded for my lack of organisation or slowness. This alternated with short-term charity jobs where I was passed up for promotion or contract renewal in favour of my white colleagues. As well as numerous unfulfilling seasonal retail and admin jobs I was completely unsuited for.

It didn't matter how hard I worked to compensate for my challenges, or my enthusiasm/loyalty to the job (which I later realised was just exploited by organisations, especially charities), my many creative ideas; or how late I stayed behind at the office after most had left. Instead all I gained was the increasing accumulation of sick days, sleepless nights, panic attacks and long cycles of burnout and recovery.

At the same I was struggling to be in healthy intimate relationships or feel secure or valued in my friendship groups. Social media only confirmed how far behind I felt compared to my peers with the seemingly linear acceleration of successful careers, serious relationships, and busy social lives.

If only I had gotten the right care, ADHD medication, therapy, self-knowledge leading to compassion, I needed before hitting adulthood. Perhaps then I could have felt less helpless, worthless and suicidal. Maybe those neural pathways wouldn't have become so set to a familiar cycle of vicious self-recrimination and crushing shame.

I really can't blame my mother too much then for thinking that a three-day self-development course could get me out of this black hole.

Five years lost to Landmark

That course was the *Landmark Forum*, the start of an elaborate pyramid scheme, run by the *Landmark Education.* A cult I later realised, whose goal was to keep you in their never-ending series of Large Group Awareness Training (LGAT) courses.[23] Once fully in, you ended up volunteering (or 'assisting' as they called it) very long hours (equivalent to a part-time job) to recruit new members, all apparently for your own 'growth' but really for their financial benefit.

Landmark achieves the above by using coercive control (aka 'brainwashing') techniques, similar to Scientology, such as long indoctrination sessions complete with guided regression, NLP and hypnotherapy exercises and verbal abuse and 'coaching' by a totalitarian all-knowing 'leader' (channelling the toxic masculinity and narcissism of their founder Werner Erhard). We were manipulated into imbibing dogmatic aphorisms designed to prevent critical thought. All of which helped to instil fears of ever progressing outside the cult, no matter how gruelling it got.

The influencing techniques that cults use in their early stages also work by making you feel wanted and giving you, as Robert Cialdini says 'instant friends and attention',

---

a process called 'love bombing. An addictive feeling for anyone like me looking for acceptance.

As a result of my co-dependence on this organisation, I ended up internalising Landmark's extremely harsh, individualist and neo-liberal ideology, one that prizes self-sufficiency and self-responsibility above all else. One which ignores the challenges of living in an ableist white supremacist society, because anything bad that happens is *all our fault*. Literally.

They are also extremely anal about lateness because, being even a few minutes late means you have to 'restore integrity' to a room full of smug punctual people if you arrive even a few minutes late. Just imagine what that does to someone who already has so much shame about their tardiness.

I was once verbally abused by a Landmark seminar leader for being 15 minutes late. He shouted at me so aggressively in front of others, that I was driven to tears. I was the one who had to apologise. Being late still leads to a rapid disintegration of my self-esteem today.

Another time I had a glimpse into the lethal nature of Landmark's techniques on mentally vulnerable people, when I had to listen to a woman on the telephone telling me that their female partner had killed themselves due to being 'triggered' on the Forum.

I was lucky. But I was left with long-term trauma - probable exacerbated CPTSD, bouts of rage and deep depression, guilt at how I manipulatively tried to recruit people, shame at my Autistic naivete and a deep sense of betrayal.

Maybe I would've understood earlier the socio-economic barriers I faced and had better self-compassion if I hadn't ended up here. Maybe I would've got my diagnosis earlier, instead of hoping this cult could 'fix' me…

My self-diagnosis

When I chanced upon my ADHD diagnosis through an accidental Google search on how to stop losing things in 2016, it was a paradigm-shifting moment.
I could finally have some compassion for myself.

I found my peers - the outsiders like me who struggled daily to survive in a competitive and insensitive society obsessed with the ideas of 'success', 'professionalism' and 'productivity' (reminds me of this cult I was in…). They understood what it was like to feel judged for failing to act like a 'real adult', observe weird social rules, or have a 'five-year plan' (does anyone actually have one of these!?).

Finding activists in the Neurodiversity movement and especially those who were also multiply-marginalised or didn't have to be given a 101 education on what racism is (beware those majority-white support groups who have a 'no politics' policy, which basically translates to 'please don't talk about your identity issues if you're marginalised because that's well awks for us and we're all equal here aren't we?'), was when true healing could begin.

But I still craved the validation and certainty of a diagnosis and access to medication that could make a substantial difference to my exhaustingly chaotic existence.

Little did I know how hard that would be…

Neo-liberal mental healthcare

I am based in Camden, supposedly one of the best boroughs in London for mental health. Even here, an

ADHD referral can lead to waiting lists of up to five years with no recourse to a shorter waiting list.

Even before that, there are huge barriers in getting referred by GPs who are largely ignorant and/or suspicious about ADHD as a valid diagnosis, especially when you add in the fact of having a marginalised identity.

When I at first, nervously, approached my GP and presented my diligently filled-in ADHD self-report scale and findings. The first thing they said with a patronisingly concerned tone was, 'are you sure it isn't anxiety, the medication is pretty heavy?' Another GP would only offer anti-depressants for my anxiety - impatient and frustrated with my insistence on an ADHD referral, telling me I should just be 'grateful' for what I could get.

In the interim, I took up another GP's offer of a referral to IAPT sessions consisting of six 30-minute identikit sessions (most of which I turned up late for so were actually 20 minutes...). There were lots of printouts, mindfulness/CBT exercises and strongly suggested recommendations for generic workshops ('why don't you try the one on anxiety?').

The whole experience made me feel like I was living in a vacuum, with the focus on what *you* can do to think more positively and basically stop being such an economic drain. Not surprising given that the use of CBT was originally marketed as a cost-saving measure...

The inaccessibility of diagnosis

Fed up with getting nowhere on the NHS, I got a private diagnosis in January 2018. Although my relief at finally being vindicated with an ADHD diagnosis was palpable, it cost nearly £600 at the time to do so (it's almost twice that now). Further appointments combined with medication prescriptions cost another £270 per month.

Meanwhile, the therapist I had found, one of the only ones I *could find* who knew anything about ADHD, but appeared to know nothing about racism, cost £65 a week. The only way I could afford all this was via the generous bank of mum and dad.

Many multiply-marginalised neurominorities I know could never afford this. Many are also estranged from families who fail to recognise their disability or accept them. Many probably don't even make it to even self-diagnosis, let alone diagnosis.

Whilst having middle-class privileges and some social skills can also lead to disadvantages in getting diagnosed. Having an MA, being social, articulate, and able to hold some eye contact i.e., mask, meant I'm often told 'but you don't look autistic!' People like me are more likely to be diagnosed with depression, anxiety or BPD. And if you're a racialised AMAB and/or poor you could even be sectioned as schizophrenic and violently psychotic.[24]

This issue is compounded by the stereotypical presentations of autism and neurodivergence in mainstream media, starting with *The Rain Man* (1988) and extending to TV series like *The Big Bang Theory* (2006) and *The Good Doctor* (2017) *etc.*, making it even harder for people like me to self-identify or be recognised as having AuDHD before even getting to referral.

As someone who isn't a mathematical/scientific savant etc (I have probable dyscalculia for one…), I can only think that this influenced how long it took for the medical system to understand my challenges.

By the time the AQ10 assessment came up as part of my NHS ADHD assessment in 2019, I had self-diagnosed with autism after extensive research, prompted by my partner

---

[24] https://www.openaccessgovernment.org/black-autism/91621/

and an AuADHD acquaintance. The Samantha Craft list[25] of autistic female traits provided further confirmation. So, when it came to passing the test, I thought I could quite easily pass...

My first red flag was when the assessor, an apparently award winning 'neurodivergent specialist nurse' started asking leading questions such as, 'You don't collect things do you?'. It left me angry and upset that he could so blatantly skew the assessment with foregone conclusions, despite all my thorough research.

Surprise, surprise. I didn't pass the test.

The problematic AQ10

Further problems emerge when examining the AQ10 tool itself, devised by Simon Baron-Cohen and his team at Cambridge. The tool only tests four supposedly common autistic traits related to things like social and behavioural challenges and limited interests. All of which are based on Baron-Cohen's disproved but sadly still prevalent, neurosexist and pathologising theories like his idea that autism originates in 'extreme male brains' and we're basically just pattern seeking sociopaths (See his 'theory of mind' and ideas on 'zero empathy').

It is infuriatingly simplistic (don't you just love government-implemented cost-saving measures already), only allowing you to 'agree or disagree' to SBC's binary, white heteronormative ideas about autism. Neither does it control for co-occurring neurodivergent conditions like ADHD (shockingly co-occurrence of ADHD and ASD wasn't recognised by the DSM until 2013).

---

[25]   http://www.myspectrumsuite.com/samantha-crafts-autistic-traits-checklist/

Take the extremely vague statement 'I find it difficult to work out people's intentions'. What if my perceptions are informed by over a decade of feeling betrayed by white liberals with so-called 'good intentions', who then proceed to bully and racelight you?

'Agreeing' to try and score high enough on this absurdly reductive test would be denying my own reality, compounding my sense of epistemic homelessness. Ultimately it seemed to me, a re-traumatising zero sum game.

What next?

After this awful assessment experience, the next viable route was to complain and try to fight for the opportunity to fill in the A50 (the longer version of the A10).

However, my detailed complaint was patronisingly almost completely dismissed by Camden & Islington Foundation Trust. I was even told that the assessors' leading questions were a result of the 'direct and specific questions' of the AQ10 tool and not because of their 'personal approach to questioning'(WTF!?).

Another bureaucratic door slammed in my face. I couldn't help thinking they *knew* they were just doing some institutional gaslighting/racelighting, but they needed to try and shut me up somehow.

You cannot cut corners and hope to capture the large variety of autistic people like me who don't live up to simplistic stereotypes, especially when those assessment methods are fuelled by white supremacist thinking.

This bias needs to be urgently, consciously identified and unlearned. But with the pace the NHS moves at and the

Overton window so far to the right, decolonisation isn't likely to happen anytime soon.

'Not autistic enough'

I finally completed the AQ50 form, only after numerous, frequent complaints and references to the Equality Act, and sent it in with a supporting evidence form completed by my mum. But for all that effort I still apparently didn't 'score high enough' to qualify for an assessment.

As a direct result of autistic naivete, ironically, I believed that my answers would be enough, not realising that I needed to have guided my mum's answers. There was no consideration for a mother's lack of awareness around autism, or the biases of a Zimbabwean immigrant/refugee whose trauma marred their ability to recognise or acknowledge my challenges.

So many like me would've easily given up at this stage, filled with self-doubt about the accuracy of their self-diagnosis, as I was at the beginning of my awareness. Drained (especially with our heightened sensitivities) by this hollowed-out process with no humanity and 'zero empathy'.

I was just lucky to find someone with some understanding left in the rigid NHS system, who accepted my mum's perspective may have been 'biased' and agreed to me submitting another form. This was over year ago at time of writing, I still haven't done it.

The more I go through this process, the more I think what's the point? Do I have it in me to fight this catch-22 system that's stacked against the most marginalised, or abandon my core beliefs of being honest and authentic trying to game a robotic system?

We urgently need targeted support for marginalised neurodivergent academics, psychologists, psychiatrists and therapists and more independent oversight of the NHS. We need more intersectional neurodivergent peer-lead training for *all* frontline staff and to value lived experience expertise by training and paying more neurodivergent peer supporters over unqualified gatekeepers; so-called 'experts' whose role seems to be excluding access to vital support, because someone doesn't fit their narrow criteria or ignorant presumptions.

Ultimately, I know that we need to try and make society a more accepting and safer place to live for *everyone*, regardless of cognitive difference and that can start with better, more nuanced media representation...

We need more compassion and understanding of how difficult and scary it can be to talk to your GP or even a loved one about your mental health, let alone a neurological condition that is so badly misunderstood.

I am grateful for this opportunity to tell *my* story which I recognise as a privilege and hope that it speaks to those queerdos unable, for whatever reason, to currently tell theirs. You're not alone.

12

ACTS OF WILL - S. Kraftowitz

A toast
For all our messy parts
  Mazeltov and welcome
                    Loosen, make yourself soft and
clear.

                    Breathe with me?

Hello. I'm Saskia and as a teenager I received anorexia treatment in hospital. Down the corridor from my mum while she was dying of cancer. I was 14 years old with emerging questions about my relationship to Jewish heritage and queerness. My mother was diagnosed with stage 4 cancer. At the same time, I was developing dysfunctional eating habits - I understood later this was a way of navigating my relationship with my intersecting identities. My mum lived for 10 months, two weeks of which we shared in hospital together.

Wrong thing to do. Am I ready to tell this story? I haven't even told it to
    myself. That's not really true. It feels quite intense. That's okay.

Here I'm sharing three acts of will. By this I mean, self-generated interventions I made in hospital to reframe my relationship to food and eating. I acted to redeem a sense of agency in the face of a stubborn medical system which could only characterise me as anorexic. Each of the actions I made was a vital glimmer of empowerment; harvesting sweet cherries growing in the hospital garden against my daily food plan, requesting and feeding beetroot soup to my mum just before her death and asking for silent, private space to wash and cleanse her body at the hospice - *Tahara.*

All three provided creative, redemptive relief in a hospital that didn't know how to cater to the nuance of my identity. With my chapter I will explore each as a pivotal happening on my journey through life. Calling this 'survival' doesn't feel quite right, because I am still affected by these events and I'm okay with that. What happened is beyond my control but I am not a victim of the world, so I am calling this my ongoing story. Acts of ritual healing have emerged from my madness, because madness itself is the symptom and the cure. Through my actions, I found pleasure that was specific to my body and identity. A radical kind of pleasure that reclaimed my autonomy and self-hood as separate from the perspective of NHS medical treatment.

Madness is a gift.
Where my madness makes others uncomfortable
I know no shame.

Notice reflective notes interjecting from the right hand side? They are insights from the personal journal I kept as I struggled to write my chapter, which I have kept. Each was an anthem in the face of difficulty. Writing this brought a challenge of physical restlessness which I have hemmed into the text, so that author and reader can move together. Follow my notes to embody the journey with me. I want to connect with you however possible as I share my story.

Pay as much attention to these as you find pleasurable.

Beginnings

Much of the anxiety about my identity was about *hidden difference*. Being Jewish, and having faced anti-semitism at school I felt there was a secret in my skin.

My socialisation had told me to keep hidden. I'm accustomed to assimilating, and veiling my truth. For instance; my family changed its name from Kraftowitz to Craft at the border. I would hide my Star of David necklace in school. Or, my attempt to play straight, despite my queerness. I grew up as an indirect descendent of genocide, and the anxiety of being visibly Jewish was reinforced by widespread incidents of anti-semitism through my teenhood. When school exposed us to explicit images of concentration camps, as we learned the detailed horrors of the Holocaust in history and RE, I struggled to cope. Friends bantered cruelly that Kraftowitz (the name I had just discovered) sounded like 'crafty bitch'. One day someone called me Anne Frank in a drama improvisation, suggesting a rape scene featuring me. It felt glamorous for a moment. Remembering it now makes me feel murderous. Recalling the memories, I see the vast white noise of my struggle with gender and body image fusing with antisemitism.

Punch. Scream. Start a fire

I hadn't lived the horrors we learned at school. Still, I despaired. I learned about Jewish history in a mostly white British non-Jewish environment and was disrespected, and unsupported through those exposures. These were the only references to Jewishness that I experienced outside the home. *Thin* and *incarcerated* became my identifiers for Judaism, easy to find in textbooks and in holocaust nostalgia media. Those images stuck around as ideas for me to idealise and replay. What I saw became a cultural wound for me to be frightened of.

There is no talk of Jews here. Jewish talk is avoided. Are Jews real? Is British Jewishness an identity negative? I know I am Jewish because I am told I shouldn't be. Jewishness feels avoided and avoidable. But I'm still here.

Starvation is a wound that can echo through generations of mental health disorder everywhere, and it is part of Jewish history. It's a fundamental aspect of my madness.

Being so thin I almost felt I could reclaim my bones. Poking through the surface of my body, I saw DNA, ancient code, the storytellers script wound in a helix. I almost reclaimed those wretched moments of history

grooving and wriggling

from a dark desire to inflict the same suffering on myself. It was perversely comforting. And who else has done this?

There's too much false hope in MH survivors giving glossy accounts of heroic recovery. I'm not interested in being a victim of romance or fetishisation.

It's only recently that I've been able to get anywhere near talking about these events in detail. Writing my chapter of Birdsong returned me to the understanding that storytelling is the fabric of my world. Finding words for this allowed me to believe that the naming of something is the healing of it. As I go, I recall the many creative outlets I've depended on to recognise and feel a part of my past. Stephen Sondheim embeds a lyric in his musical *Into The Woods* that goes 'be careful the tale you tell, that is the spell'. Just after my mum died these words told me that what I believe can become my reality. But that lyric has more wizardry to it. Tales are spells because they are *both question and answer.* Similarly, Jewish tradition has *Midrash (מדרש), '*an interpretive act, seeking the answers to religious questions (both practical and theological) by plumbing the meaning of the words of the Torah'. To protect its culture from erasure, Judaism uses critical practice. Retellings help retain the integrity of culture and heritage. Constantly investigating ideas and beliefs also allows challenging ideas to be investigated. I am seeing this chapter as an act of midrash, helping me eight years later to author a personal narrative that begins to make some more sense of this experience.

Through my years, and over the time I have been writing this chapter, I've had to extract any explanations or apologies for my madness which find their way into text. If not, I might get stuck inside the wrong person's language.

One. cherries

Close eyes. Three deep breaths. Open eyes. Feel pulses as tides.

My brother has always been a helping hand in mischief. One day I pointed to some cherries growing in the courtyard beside my mum's in-patient room, which I craved to taste. He nodded, and we picked them. At the time I had to travel everywhere by wheelchair so we sped the entire way back to my ward. My bedside observations happened three times a day and we were running late. I didn't care much. But my treatment involved draconian itineraries of eating, resting, testing. With my brother's help we stashed the cherries (there was a fridge in mum's cancer ward), except one which I hid up my sleeve. I luxuriously devoured mine in the shower, which was policed by an observation doctor who had been placed there to ensure I didn't secretly exercise.

I was acutely opposed to being a 'good-patient'. Still, I struggle sometimes to resist the trap of playing 'good' to feel safe.

As an inpatient I couldn't bear constraint. The treatment of anorexia is that you are forced into patterns of life, of eating and embodying, that are not your own. You are denied your identity and forced to adopt another one, a pathologisation. For me there was a parallel between this restriction and so many aspects of Jewish experience. Thoughtful support was so vitally needed in helping me process my feelings, but totally unavailable. Yet, entwined within my dysfunctional eating was my perception that my Jewish identity was irrelevant.

Picking those cherries was a way of claiming *my* hunger, and distinguishing it from conditioned eating patterns. I was recognising hunger as a signpost of existential desire, signalling the will to live and thrive. Food was my primary hunger, because it underpinned the impulse to survive. Biblically, food is the meeting point between spirit and matter. To *eat* is to enter fully into the world. It is to encounter otherness. When Eve eats the apple, she takes it in. I desperately needed to re-engage with the sensuality and spiritedness of eating, to eat as a way to understand the otherness of everything... of myself, of the world.

My memory of picking cherries carries a curious parallel to the biblical idea of Eden. Someone had thought to plant a beautiful garden in the precinct of the oncology ward, and no one else was picking the perfectly ripe cherries there. They were rotting in the burning sunshine. It was no longer any part of the medical establishment. This is partly why what I did was transgressive. I accessed what felt like a hidden treasure. More than that, though, it was forbidden; it wasn't in my eating plan, the fruit was hanging in the garden of the ward where my mum was dying. What I recognised in my desire to pick those cherries was a reclamation of spiritual entwinement with eating.

Look 20 feet into the distance and then come back.

I encountered my emerging sexuality in that action. To eat the cherries was to say yes to survival, to being alive, to desire and therefore to having a sexuality. A sexuality. That was also transgressive for me as I am queer. At the time of my greatest dysfunctionality with eating, I was quite unable to articulate why I was so conflicted about having sexuality. As an adult I can clearly understand how threatening the concept was. Being a young assigned-female body at puberty required endurance. I was confronted by my queerness while also repelled by how hurtful the objectification of my mature body might be.

Two.

Beetroot soup

My mother and I were in the hospice, days from the end of her life. She was struggling to eat, despite the care team trying to offer her appealing food. Because of the stent in her colon, she had to eat smooth, un-irritating food, which she'd done since diagnosis. For both of us I wished for a more free and beautiful experience of being ill. When I noticed the visitor cafe serving beetroot soup, I caught an incredible opportunity to bring mum joy. After nurses swapped her lunch routine, the two of us alone did lunch. Spoon by spoon I slowly fed her, observing affectionately in case she didn't like it or needed to stop. She couldn't speak or communicate much at this point and had everything done for her. I smiled across the plastic tray while she made small sounds.

howl I don't know if I'm crying or laughing or crying

Being in hospital shifted the dynamic for mum and I. Our usual family bonds were transformed, queered even, by our context. We were levelled; equally patients, both with illnesses relating to food, both depersonalised individuals in the same hospital. Our proximity to death warped the etiquette of parent-child bond and we began to care for each other reciprocally. When I had snuck into mum's ward, we took turns looking after each other, putting on a film, making tea, running showers, giving the other what we could not have for ourselves. Feeding my mum restored our conviviality. I wanted so much for us to exist in space together, breathe together. Where illness altered our connection, hospital care exacerbated it with a rigid system that barely allowed us to see each other, that absolutely couldn't make space for our grief. What is the appropriate response when a family is dying? What is the measure of emotional vs medical need?

———

Grief can go somewhere. It can dance through our lives. *Dancing Grooving*

Whenever I look back on the memory it is drenched with colour. I can see a bowl of red, mirroring the blood which bound us. Something about the centrality of care and feeding in a Jewish parent-child relationship was important for me to recover, even if it had to happen the wrong way around. Food is written into the mythic narrative of Judaism, it's everywhere in the rules, ceremony, celebration. As a group of diasporic people who move unpredictably, food is a reliable domestic ritual. Meals provide a sense of meaning, identity and safety. Understanding that food could not be ritualised, or encultured in my treatment, or mums, stole my joy. In a

medical context, eating becomes dry and scientific. Picking cherries, feeding beetroot soup to my mother; they were both ways to nourish our sense of self. It is so heartbreaking to share a last supper with a loved one. Watching their last breath even feels whimsical and fleeting, by comparison.

More memories come, short exhales...

me and mum stealing food from Bat Mitzvah and kiddush tables. our handbags

overflowing with Challah and boiled eggs. great garlands of fruit stretched across a towering sukkah. me scampering to find hidden bread followed by mum's wide almond eyes. long blue evenings dipping herbs in salty water, recounting the tale of pesach.

breathe all the air out.

Three. Tahara.

There was never any attempt from psychiatry or my anorexia treatment to talk about bodies, it was always about eating. This still shocks me. My struggle to *be* my body wasn't being picked up by healthcare. One single instance when I was assigned space to talk, I felt incredibly unsafe. The Jewishness of my body was invisible. My gender was assumed. I was terrified to grow into a body which would be gendered, objectified and sexualised by the world. Even worse was to remain silent.

Food restriction is a common and effective puberty blocker in the queer community which I called on to cope. Without dysfunctional eating it felt unworkable to navigate how I related with gender and what that meant for my body, and even more to be a Jewish body. Becoming a *thin body* provided scope to protect and consider my vulnerability. Across the years of in and out-patient treatment I received, there was no sense that the somatic needed to be tended. It was disappointing that my treatment would locate the problem in my head, or on my plate. Which is where washing my mum's dead body came in. My aunt, my grandmother and I gathered a few hours after my mum died, to cleanse and prepare her for burial. It is a Jewish tradition called Tahara.

Tahara cleanses and sacralises a body for death, but what was important for me in this moment was that I got to sacralise the marginality. The severity of mum's illness caused her to balloon and distend. My body looked like a glass animal. Un-ideal body shape became holy under our hands. As I sponged mum's delicate skin, I wanted to inhabit it. Ceremony helped me honour a Jewishness which rooted through her muscle and bone. A door opened for me then, to invite in the Jewishness of my own body, whenever I choose.

Mum, with her domed belly, almost looked pregnant. On the threshold of her life ending, mine metamorphosed adopting a new form. Encountering otherness by seeing mum's dead body, became a way for me to understand how peculiar and fundamentally changing a human is from start to end. The transition of a body's shape can be colossal from a gender perspective. Weaving through my considerations of gender was a sense of burgeoning Jewish embodiment. At the time I was close to a common coming of age ritual where I might have 'grown' in all senses into my Jewishness. Queerness answers this kind of moment with the perspective that as a queer person grows to realise their identity there is death and rebirth which repeats whenever necessary. We worked over the whole body and I felt new. As I sponged mum's delicate skin, I

wanted to inhabit it. Instead I grew through and from the moment. Washing her was profoundly human and normal. Her body was my body, it was other, it was un-idealised, it was dead.

up all night, talking, talking, reading the Kaddish aloud, listening to Ray Charles blues shout blind on the phonograph

the rhythm the rhythm—and your memory in my head three years after—And read Adonais' last triumphant stanzas aloud—wept, realizing how we suffer—

Kaddish - Allen Ginsberg, 1961

At that moment Jewish ritual gave me a promise that our bodies, no matter what, are beautiful. To wash mum was to admit that she was divine, and to hold her journey to death in a way that was sacred.

No psychiatry, no treatment, no medical context would have had the transformative power which that moment offered me. Tahara was simple poetry. And it has only ever been poetry - necessary and inevitable poetry - that can answer to pain or suffering or great madness.

Hug your body.

To End

_____

Madness wants to be understood as more than its symptoms. All of my actions, from picking cherries to washing mum's body, I did to rehumanise myself. Everything in the context of my hospital treatment had been narrowed down and I became only 'a person with anorexia'. The failure and distress in the care I received, is that it denied me the opportunity to be anything other than a textbook case. What my interventions always tried to do was to give me a sense of being much more than that. Writing here and accessing ongoing help from the right places has shown me the world is large enough to hold me.

Wanting fluidity but afraid of gendered body expectations, fondly admiring my Judaism but ashamed of its public image, shattered by the imminent loss of my mum; Madness, for me, blasted simplicity and drew together each fold of my worries. Starved-body holocaust images, tiny-sexualised-objectified-gendered bodies, Mum who literally looked like a dying thing, and *me* resembling a little of each.

Mine is an odd and beautiful existence. My me-ness encompasses my madness, gender, sexuality, being Jewish and the life-altering effects of bereavement. I unlearn, relearn and new-learn like I am dreaming. Amongst the chaos, my body was and will always be a site of primary agency. Eating is a way to inhabit my life, to cross and know its land.

13

TREADING WATER - C Biln

I need to set a scene to help me share things with you. It's highly likely that I'm going to have a mug of peppermint tea cradled in my hands. You'll ask me how I've been and, after a deep breath, I'll say that I should probably start at the beginning.

One thing you should know first is that I like to *compartmentalise*. I'm aware that everything in life weaves together in wild and wonderful ways, however, in order for me to make sense of things, I have to section off parts of myself and the world around me. If you feel that something is missing or left unsaid, it's because I can only focus on one issue at a time.

My Teens

I cannot pinpoint exactly when I started to notice issues with my mental health. It wasn't until my mid-twenties that I started to truly learn about mental illness so I guess I was unaware of things prior to that. What I do know is that I was very morbid in my teens. Most of my time was divided between considering my own death and the deaths of others. When I thought about my death, I would list how it would benefit those around me, how I was worthless and how I was making everyone else miserable. When I thought about others, I wondered how they would die and how I would not be able to survive without them. As much as I wanted to, I could never stop thinking about this.

Along with these gloomy thoughts, I had a tendency to self-harm, binge eat, isolate myself and obsess over how I looked. For the most part, I thought this was just part and parcel of being a teenager – I'd grow out of it at some point.

It wasn't until my parents split up when I was in sixth form that I spoke to someone outside my immediate family about my bleak thoughts. Through her work, my mum was able to get me six free counselling sessions so for one hour a week I could open up to someone honestly. Much of the counselling was beneficial: I learned about setting boundaries, being kinder to myself, communicating honestly and listening actively. The hardest struggle was trying to work out why anything mattered if, ultimately, we were all going to die anyway. In response to my question, my counsellor suggested that we can exist to improve the lives of others and make them happy. While that piece of advice helped to pull me out of my downward morbid spiral, it also started my painful addiction to people-pleasing.

For about a year, I thought I'd cracked it. I'd done all right in my A-levels, got into a good university and found a solid friendship circle. The problem was that even though things weren't as bad, my fears were still present in the background every day. At nineteen, I finally decided to talk to my doctor. I remember saying that I was feeling really down and I couldn't stop thinking horrible things. The doctor was typing on his computer as I was talking. He turned to me and said that a lot of people feel like this in their teens and it'd sort itself out over time. He then weighed me and said I was obese and if I lost some weight, I would feel better.

My Twenties

With this message planted firmly in my head, I went to Germany to work as a language assistant for a year. It was my first time away from home and I was quite isolated in a small German village where I stuck out like a sore thumb, both aesthetically and linguistically. I had friends dotted around the country but I would frequently spend weekends on my own. During this period, I developed very obsessive behaviours which significantly impacted my life. Every week, I would buy the same basket of shopping and eat the exact same food on the exact same day unless I had a visitor. I developed a fear about wetting myself in public so I went to the toilet religiously every hour – if I couldn't, I would not stop thinking about it until I finally got to a loo. Walking was something I could lose myself in so I would walk for miles and miles for no reason. When I was on my own, I steadily ate less and less, prodding my increasingly-prominent bones on a nightly basis. I'm still not sure why I did this but on reflection I now think I was struggling with all of the changes that had taken place and that the only real control I had was over my food and my body. Over the year, I lost a significant amount of weight.

When I came home, my obsessions stayed with me. My family noticed straight away, through my extreme mood swings and compulsive behaviours. Looking back now, I'm aware that I was very difficult to live with. Even though they cared, I pushed everyone's concerns away and threw myself back into my studies. After my previous experience with my doctor, why would I subject myself to discomfort and dismissal again?

For roughly seven years, I coped like this through graduation, my PGCE and the start of my teaching career. During this time, I experienced panic attacks, further disordered eating, bouts of incredibly low mood and anxiety. I masked this all the time in professional spaces and brought my difficult feelings back home where I took them out on the people I loved and myself.

It got particularly bad in my fourth year of teaching. I hit a point where I didn't want to die – I just didn't want to exist. My obsession with diet, exercise and how I looked was at an all-time high. I was having panic attacks on a daily basis. I struggled to sleep. It was getting harder and harder to mask how I was feeling at work. My husband pushed me to talk to my doctor (a new one) about what I was going through. After one long, intense and heart-wrenching conversation, I was diagnosed with anxiety. I was not happy.

No-one in my family has ever spoken much about mental health – we had other concerns in life. When I found out about my anxiety, I also found out that I couldn't make it all disappear in an instant. In fact, my anxiety diagnosis made me more anxious – how was I going to deal with this great unknown? My doctor offered me pills, talking therapies and a note to be signed off from work. I felt so much shame even at the idea of being away from my work structure. I'd worked hard to build my teaching career and I didn't want it to be marred by having mental illness on my records. After overhearing conversations between my family members and at work, I gathered that pills had a lot of stigma attached to them – I didn't want to have people think less of me for needing a mental crutch.

In the end, I went for talking therapies and a lifestyle change (changing my job so I had short walk to work rather than a long commute on public transport). While I wasn't the biggest fan of the CBT and one-to-one discussions (I was in such a mental and emotional mire that I didn't understand how anything suggested was relevant to my situation), I slowly found strategies that helped me overcome a lot of my issues. My relationship with food and exercise became more balanced, I got out of the house more and I had fewer and fewer panic attacks. It didn't mean my mental health issues completely disappeared; I had to monitor how I was feeling and my behaviours on a regular basis. From time to time, I had flare-ups but at least now I had strategies to help me catch myself before it got particularly bad. I felt like I was getting into a good headspace.

My Thirties

Then, tragically, my grandma passed away in 2019. It was something my family knew was going to happen but it hit us hard nonetheless. I was signed off work for three weeks, mainly to support my mum and because I was so exhausted. I'd never experienced the death of a family member before so I didn't know what to expect. My grandpa's house was constantly full of people, many of whom I barely knew or had never met before.

On a near daily basis, we spent a long time cooking for lots of people. I was faced with a number of cultural matters I'd never encountered before: men eating before women, no meat in the house, kava drinking sessions and doing absolutely everything your elders ask of you. It was a shock to the system, especially as I'd lived with my grandparents for three years during university and I thought I knew them pretty well.

Just six weeks later, I was told my estranged father had also died. It was all a blur. Even though I had time off, I never had the much-needed quiet time to grieve. Before I knew it, I had a three-week phased return to work and then I was back to teaching full-time. It wasn't easy but thankfully I knew ways to support my mental health which enabled me to cope.

The following September, I moved to a new school to take on some different challenges. This time, I properly opened up to my family, friends and co-workers about my mental health, less fearful of the stigma and aware that I needed some external help as my grief was still quite raw. Opening up had a really positive impact on my first year: I felt comfortable enough to talk freely and I didn't have to mask my feelings all the time. My confidence as a teacher grew and I began to have much more work-life balance.

The Pandemic

Then Covid hit in March 2020, setting into motion a whole mess of problems. I lost my routine, my support network and my mental escapes but I continued in my role as a key worker through each and every lockdown. I genuinely thought I was coping tremendously well. I didn't have any breakdowns or panic attacks, I created my own routines and I threw myself into work.

Looking back, I realise that I really wasn't processing what was going on and didn't want to think about it so I filled my life with work (even when I didn't need to). From professional development courses to planning, I focused on my role as teacher as the rest of me faded away.

From spring 2020 onwards, my work-life balance vanished, as did all my ability to disconnect myself from my key worker role. This was not only evident in my day-to-day tasks but also in my self-care: I struggled with personal hygiene, putting on clean clothes, getting enough sleep, talking to my doctor and accessing my usual tried-and-tested self-help strategies for anxiety. I blamed much of what I was experiencing on the pandemic, my essential job and people's expectations of me. I felt like I couldn't take a breath or pause because, if I did, I wouldn't be doing my job properly, I'd let everyone down and then everyone would hate me. I know now that this was an awful negative spiral but at the time, it was all I could focus on.

In September 2021, a co-worker found me crying in my classroom and suggested I have a chat to my doctor. I was so livid that I exploded – I did not believe that I needed to talk to anyone because I knew my options and nothing would help. Two months later, after increasing spells of low mood and a few big panic attacks, I was signed off work for a month. I was beside myself. Unlike my previous experience of grief, there was no big life-changing event or tragedy: this time it was just me. Guilt and fear ate away at me and I told myself every horror story I'd imagined about my life was going to come true. I was forced to pause and, while the daily stress of teaching disappeared, my difficult feelings, wild fears and paranoia remained and sadly grew. I hit a point where I thought everyone in my life was against me and I was going to lose my job.

The Here and Now

As this has all been so recent, I haven't been able to properly reflect and work out what actually sparked the beginnings of my recovery.

Reading has always been a source of comfort for me and I read a lot while I was signed off, focusing on issues like burnout, managing anxiety and prioritising tasks. I then used my new-found knowledge to add in some helpful strategies to my self-care. Friends have been honest during conversations and I've been able to talk through my feelings without judgement. Doing this has helped me to uncover issues I've been unaware or ignorant of. Instead of starting each day considering hundreds of different boxes I need to tick, I just focus on one or two which has had a huge impact on my mental load and exhaustion. Talking to my doctor made a huge difference too, I am lucky enough to be able to see someone who is able to be both empathetic and assertive regarding my mental health needs. In turn, being slowly supported back into teaching has helped me reconnect with the joy in my job. Rather than seeing teaching as my sole purpose in life, it's now just an element of my existence.

In The Background

While all this has been going on, I have existed as a woman of colour in majority white spaces: from student to teacher, from supermarket customer to book club member, from service user to friend. Every day of my life, I am in the minority – unless I'm with my family. This alone takes a toll on my general wellbeing.

When considering the intersection between my mental health and my race, I can identify two major issues. Firstly, I do not see people who look like me talk about mental health, and neither do I see people like me experience similar issues such as isolation or grief.

Much of what I am and have been exposed to in popular culture, medical literature, social media and beyond is generally focused on white women. I have had to dig and research to find reflections of myself in the world of mental illness. This also means that medical professionals and people in general don't necessarily associate brown faces with mental health issues. In my experience, this means that my concerns aren't always taken seriously and I have to push for more. Moreover, while my family background and my culture aren't the most prominent elements of my day-to-day, there are issues and experiences I deal with that the white majority is completely ignorant of: the constant feeling of not fitting in anywhere, people querying my heritage and stereotyping among many others. Because of this, it can be difficult to talk about issues with professionals who are unaware of the impact of lived experience. When you have to do the intellectual and emotional labour of conveying this, it can lead to often uncomfortable conversations that are hard to navigate. Not only does this make you feel tired and irritable, but after a while it wears you down and you wonder why you bothered in the first place. This results in a struggle to find the right support without experiencing additional trauma.

Additionally, mental illness is not really talked about in my South Asian culture. My immediate family has become more open over the years but it's not always easy. One family member is well-meaning but often queries what has been the cause of my mental health issues historically and I don't want to engage in those discussions. Older generations and those outside my close circle can be very dismissive of mental illness: sometimes people get laughed at, sometimes people are linked to witches or demons and sometimes they're just called 'wrong in the head'. This has meant that I can't always talk to people in my family about what is happening to me because of the shame and stigma around mental illness.

These two issues together have made my personal experience of mental illness tougher because I feel isolated from both my own culture and society in general. In order to gain some respite and perspective, I try to compartmentalise myself into 'South Asian me' and 'mental health me'. However, I'm aware that considering myself in this way is not workable in the long term because ultimately, the two parts influence and impact each other.

Reflection

When I think about my recent crisis and my prior low points, the frustration I have - with myself - is that I knew a lot of the self-care and strategies before AND I knew what the signs of poor mental health looked like in me but I refused to see them. Even though my loved ones signposted support, I had to hit rock bottom before I sought help and I'm trying to work out why.

Managing my mental health needs feels like treading water – it's a constant effort. Dealing with further issues linked to race and culture requires even more exertion which becomes even more exhausting. This increasing fatigue means there is even more of an urge to stop kicking my legs and let the water take me. When I get tired of treading, I stop and I end up going under. I know this but still I cannot help myself because ultimately, I guess I don't want to have to put in so much work to just be 'OK'.

Knowing my history and mental health patterns, I am fully aware that I have to continue keeping my head above water because the constant effort is better than drowning.

Keep In Mind - Privilege

In everything I have been through, I must state that I have had to be proactive and assertive in order to receive support. I have also had the privilege of being part of a social circle which includes healthcare professionals, educators and those aware of pathways for mental health support. Without my approach or connections, I do not know how I might be at this moment in time but I am not particularly hopeful. It seems unfair that all of this is required (and so much more in many cases) of people when they are feeling most lost. We all need help when we're drowning.

14

LOSING IT TO FIND IT – Nina Osei Wilson

Breakdowns in relationships I've been in: romantic, non-romantic, friendships, have all been a result of what was NOT being said. Including breakdowns of relationships with my own family members, in particular my own mother.

What we choose not to say, I believe, has links to the state of mental health we are experiencing at whatever point in time it may be. For me, at one pivotal stage in my life where I was grappling with my own mental health, I decided to say nothing. I made it a personal pursuit to be mute because I felt as though I wasn't being heard. In addition to this, I hadn't quite found the words to express what I was feeling. When I attempted to, to me, they felt incoherent. Sometimes even nonsensical because I felt there were better words to verbalise what I was trying to convey.

In a sense, I just gave up. At this point I'm unsure of how effective that was in terms of working through what I was going through at the time. What I am certain of now is that through my own recovery process and talking with people that are non-judgemental, those that are brave enough to speak up about their experiences, the people I meet in my work with mental health encourage me to keep speaking up about my ongoing journey.

There is a feel on a par to freedom or, being freed of a burden when being able to share the story of a pivotal moment in my growth.

I often find myself propelled in some kind of personal pursuit, to uncover the things that people don't say. Perhaps this pursuit is personal to me due to my own ineptitude of not being able to express myself so eloquently. No window dressing, minimal waffling but delivered in a witty way that is accessible to most.

When meeting someone new, some of us have the tendency to highlight the elements of ourselves we really want people to see. With the emphasis around what someone repeatedly illuminates, sometimes outside the dark expanse of those words lies a truth that doesn't want to be seen. The shadow of ourselves. The side of ourselves that we don't want anyone to see.

I have often struggled to take things at vocal value. Visual value sometimes tells us a lot more.

In the black community, it is all too common to sweep any signs of mental distress exhibited by others and even ourselves under the carpet.

I can see this in my own family. For as long as I could remember, my mother's mental health condition didn't have a name. The time period for which my mother was at the peak of her sickness was also referred to as, 'When your mother was ill'. Quite considerate when I think of the different ways mental health conditions are usually described. Usually leaning towards a more derogatory slant. The word 'ill' could take on various forms and shapes with it being vague for an explanation.

Watching my mother, who has a longstanding history of schizophrenia following post-natal depression, ignore her sister's mental distress when she came to occupy our living room left me dumbfounded. It was wild to see my mother ridicule her own sister and shut off empathy for her situation all together.

See this is the thing, I don't think that my mother is able to adopt an 'if-the-shoe-was-on-the-other-foot' perspective at all. Completely forgetting the years and energy that my father and even her son have spent looking after her when she was severely ill.

When I first started to feel unlike myself, my first response was to get away. Similar to when I go on a night out and have too much to drink. Rather than letting those I came with see me in such a dishevelled shape, I rarely say goodbye and just disappear into the night. A similar approach was applied to my mental health difficulties initially.

My version of running away entailed going to Belgium without telling anyone until I was there. On top of this, meeting up and staying with a Nigerian guy that I had known for no more than a week. I had no family connections out there and that suited me fine: I was trying to escape on my own. Long story short, I got arrested and by the grace of the Most High, I managed to talk myself out of it.

Shortly after this incident and multiple arguments with this Nigerian guy, I knew I had to face the demons that existed on my home turf. On very little sleep and minimal food, I organised to move back into a flat, a good few stops away from my mother's house. That's where I'd been living prior to me leaving for Belgium. The very centre of my mental distress. I knew if I were to uncover brighter times, it was not going to be under my mother's roof.

To provide some much-needed context, what encouraged me to see refuge as far away from home as possible, was the ever-tumultuous relationship with my mother. I couldn't bear to be in the same room as her for a couple years. When she entered a room, I'd swiftly exit it. If I heard her voice, I had to drown it out with music via headphones or by blaring my music at maximum decibels.

But now I had to go home. I couldn't live this 'fairytale' that had morphed into a nightmare. I foresaw that trying to get my belongings from my mother would be another nightmare waiting for me on the horizon. I honestly thought that by contacting the police on the night I decided to take the plunge, I would be in safe hands…

I couldn't have been more wrong.

At first sight of the police, I suspect that my mother assumed the worst. She isn't living a squeaky-clean life and assumed that I had thrown her under the bus for her iniquities. I recall her and my boy cousin speaking in their local dialect which I don't understand. The words she spoke were: 'I haven't seen her for the whole day but I know she's been smoking weed'. These were the words she spoke to the policeman who attended.

I lost it.

Why was the truth difficult for my mother to mouth? Why did she feel it necessary to do this to me? Why did she not speak on the circumstances that pushed me away to another country with a complete stranger - our living room being occupied by her sister - who has a severe mental health condition - and unfortunately her sister's unruly son was an accompanying party? Let's not forget that I had now become a surrogate mother for my nephew. A nephew that was not going to listen to his mother, let alone me as his newly appointed surrogate. Yes, I do believe in the ethos that it takes a village or a community to raise a child. A community does not consist of one person, it's a collective effort. Although the place that was supposed to be my home was to the brim with relatives; people with opinions on what should be done, responsibility was made mine by my mother and my aunties.

Going back to the moment where the policeman showed up... A verbal battle ensued between my mother and I, which the police officer who was on scene watched for minutes on end before he decided he had enough of witnessing our dispute. I was pushed against the brick wall that housed my mother's front door; arms pushed up into an agonising position before cuffs being tightly slapped onto my wrists. I have never, to date, experienced such a sharp sensation of pain. In a frantic attempt to free myself from this situation, I called out to the white male neighbour who lives across the road. I guess my rationale behind this was the fact that he was aware of the negative impact living with my mother was having on me and my older sibling. In addition, he always seemed to have a keen interest in our family affairs and therefore I felt he was watching most of the time.

There was no response. No-one came to help.

Since the incident I vowed, even in a life-or-death situation to never contact the police for support of any kind. Non-coincidentally, any trust I had in people dissipated in a matter of minutes.

This incident occurred back in 2016, and five years on I received a half-hearted apology from my mother, likely to have been inspired by the fact that I am the one she calls for help with passport renewal, replacement gas meter cards, ongoing issues with her understanding her mobile phone. Essentially, I was carrying out administration without the respect that all administrators rightfully deserve. She couldn't even bring herself to explain what it was she was apologising for when I asked.

What would a forgivable apology look like? What would it feel like? Changed behaviour to the first. Genuine changed behaviour to both. I like to be optimistically honest: that isn't going to happen. That doesn't stop a small part of me hoping.

I haven't forgiven, nor have I forgotten. My soul tells me that it's the Most High that I regularly consult to have patience to even speak to her. Family and friends are quick to remind me that 'I only get one mother'. Yes. This is factual however, my mother has happily thrown me under the bus, refuses to recognise what she has done and STILL leans on me for my support. I can't even put into words the effect this has on the dynamic of our relationship as well as my own mental health.

I still try to do what is right in the form of helping her when I can. However, in order for me to truly own my recovery process, it is critical that I misplace my relationship with my mother in order to pursue my true callings in life - helping others that need extra support as a result of injustice, being misunderstood and or, just want someone to listen without judgement.

What that looks like to me, and has done since September 2019, is helping others that have found themselves sectioned, marginalised and isolated, all whilst trying to manage mental distress. I started off working on a 1:1 basis as a Peer Support Worker with a charity and now I currently work for the NHS with the same job title. When I first started my job as a PSW with the NHS, the focus was to obtain the untold stories of those admitted onto wards. The day-to-day discomforts that come with having your freedom taken away while being on a psychiatric ward. The importance of choice and having a say in one's own healthcare.

Now my PSW role is centred on the activities that people can undertake to help manage the difficult moments in recovery. Working on various wards, engaging with people through creative means such as music, poetry, art has allowed me to see therapy in a new light. I consider these creative therapies as essential daily occupations that I immerse myself. In coming to this realisation, I almost made a mistake in terms of my career direction, as I applied for and was accepted on an Occupational Therapy Apprenticeship. Once believing that Occupational Therapy had a subcategory for which Art Psychotherapy came under when in actuality, there are many types of creative therapies which are inclusive in Art Therapy.

For over a decade I had indulged in self-taught Photography and worked as a Freelance Photographer, unknowingly engaging in a creative therapy. It was only until my main camera lens was damaged accidentally that I felt the pangs of loss through not being able to capture on DSLR. In this long-standing interim, it has been paint, pens and paper that have filled the void. Job satisfaction looks and feels like being able to help others but also, in doing so, being able to heal my own wounds. There more I consider this perspective; my need to express myself through other mediums besides words, I started pursuing further studies and higher education opportunities in Art Psychotherapy.

15

IT MEANS FLIGHT IN LATIN - Martin Johnstone

In 2015 after experienced several traumatic or triggering events in a row, I entered what is known as a disassociated fugue state. I lost time and was found admitted to hospital in Taunton and then transferred to Banbury.

No one listened. They shared my personal information with my abuser. They ignored my obvious physical struggle. I had no voice. Eventually I was sent away after hearing 'there's nothing wrong with you'.

A year later I was in prison. I'd been medicated with the wrong drugs. I'd had 2 surgeries. I was discharged after x-rays revealed I'd swallowed razor blades.

I was lied to. Ignored. Dismissed. Humiliated.

No one listened. Around me, non-POC people were treated very differently and eventually I simply gave up. I was invisible in a system designed to put the burden of care on family I do not have.

1.

The word 'fugue' made my attachment to you flare as though a sun exploded somewhere far away enough to appear as a pinprick in my skin. Something that may be a 'sharp scratch' but actually fades having little to no impact. It is there, though. With me.

I cannot bear to bore you with my monologue (my diatribe even) about how 1 dictionary is not as good as another so I will not cite my definitions here. The normative definitions are:

F-U-G-U-E (fuga)

fyewg [noun]
musical composition in which a theme is repeated in different parts.

More interesting because it is perhaps more applicable:

F-U-G-I-T-I-V-E
fyewj-it-iv [noun]
person who flees, especially from arrest or pursuit [adjective] - *fleeing transient*

I sensed danger from an obligation or responsibility and ran to safety?
Safety. That's the word in your theory that pulls you apart and exposes you completely.

Frankly how anyone would consider running 29 miles a day for 7 days a 'safe' environment is not attached to any reality, thus the dissociative (*adjective*) element in Dr. Guruseamyi's phrase? If fugue is the noun, then her usage of 'dissociative' as a qualifier isn't as powerful.

My imagination creates something, of course: I have perhaps denied or broken an *association* with that I found dangerous enough to flee from: the god of the dead.

From experience, running 'ultra' distances (anything greater than a marathon) is an amazing antidote (*noun.* something that counteracts a poison) to reality. Its appeal is exactly that. Especially while entangled with you. While pounding out the miles, step by step, I only ever think of the next step forward and, at dark times, your face or a song we shared. These alternately lift me and drown me.

I'm going to ignore the Scorpion, the Rabbit and the God of the Dead as I expect within that tale, the repetition of my life takes shape. Perhaps it will be an opera 1 day. A fugue opera? 1 where both the musical and narrative themes repeat throughout? The text would read like a fugue.

I know, I know. I should not judge my own work. If as you say, Julie isn't real and I need an editor (perhaps you after settling into your new life?) who could wrangle me and my words sufficiently. For as much as I'd like you to do it, I'm inclined never to ask. I like to imagine you're reading my words in secret. I don't know why.

I'm equally inclined to pursue the fugal (?) nature of the narrative. In a strange way, the word *fuga* (the Latin) appeared recently. As though it was a dragonfly (*libellule*) or harmattan- consumed sun against a battleship-grey sky, as Guruseamyi played me some (J.S.) Bach. Well, someone playing a fuga, as written by Johann Sebastian.

How do I know? The same way I found you. The same way I ended up in that place. The same way I ended up in that city. The same way I ended up in that country.

The fuga gravitated towards me. Radio 3 played it 1 afternoon. They just did. As they would. So, I became unwrapped immediately and unable to hide any aspect of myself: I was like that with you, whether you saw it or not (a deliberate split). Because you were leaving and that was when I felt the closest. (Possibly. It is a new theory.)

What I have learned:

I am wrong about the narrative.

It is 1 thread and not many.

A literary fuga where my personality (gifts and afflictions included) is the repeating theme.

2.

It has been a week since I wrote those words, and I'm struck by how much thinking and consideration it takes to continue. How much energy it takes to think and consider.

I've woken up with a single tear in each eye. I've hurt my head whilst somnambulating. I felt you brush against me, which woke me while it was not as dramatic or weird as playing foreheads or kissing goodbye on a railway platform. Saying 'goodbye', of course. A major milestone in the narrative which I realise I haven't given breath to yet. No one has heard me give a name to what 'this' is.

I am undiagnosed.

I can feel it. Something is inside of me. It is warm and then hot and then cold.

When I listen to people tell me I am the love of their life, I am unconvinced.

A week later when I am not enough for them, I am perfectly calm.

A month later when they describe me as water because the closer they get the more intangible I become, I am not even listening.

When you are not enough for someone, you do not need to know why. I've not been enough for myself for so long.

This is a lover that told me they need me. That I am more than they ever expected. That their soul yearns for me. Their text messages haunt me. Their photos make me want to taste my own blood. Their constant calling to check in on me and tell me to take care hurt more than I imagined anything could.

I remember an evening we had. A meal. A talk. A dance. A moment when they told me it all felt so real. As though we were in something real. I tried to let it be a fantasy. I tried.

Eventually as the summer drew to a close, I accepted that I am nothing for them. Nothing to them. Their divorce finalised. I had served my purpose. My lover was gone.

Of course, they called. And messaged and finally got a hold of me on an obscure service attached to a social media giant. They told me that we never had enough time. They asked me to keep their letters safe.

What do I remember after reading those words?

Nothing until the young redhead woke me up and asked me to remember an address. I kept asking who lived there. She smiled and explained it didn't matter, and I was discharged. I was 200 miles from what was pretending to be home.

3.

A week after that I woke up somewhere else. Somewhere new. A man was telling me I could hear him. Another told me I was not alone. That I would be safe. A young nurse asked me who Maria was. I'm not sure what I told her. It didn't matter.

I was taken somewhere and introduced to Guruseamyi. A woman carved from marble who told me there was nothing wrong with me. Medically. It was something broken in my mind that they were interested in. I told her to speak to the person who broke it.

What did I mean? That we are responsible for how we treat people. We can never underestimate the impact we have. That words matter. That how you make someone feel is something that shouldn't be thought of as anything less than important.

As I walked out of that session wondering what my name was, I saw a man I recognised immediately. Years earlier he had been my boss's boss. He could recognise me. He could say my name in full.

I told him I remembered him. That we worked together at a large technology company in London. I reminded him of my ideas that he supported and my knowledge of markets that meant I was invited to his senior meetings. I reminded him of a success we had shared.

He smiled. He waited for me to walk away, having accepted his nodding. I realised that he did not know me. A man I had worked under. To whom I'd dedicated weekends and late nights. A man who was meant to be impressed because he was impressive. A man who guided our lives by picking slots we would fill and bonuses we would or would not be paid – he had forgotten me completely. I was right. I was nothing.

Except no one knew what was wrong with me. The question mark over my head was a sword of Damocles. What date awaited me after someone decided how I would be classified or reconciled?

I waited.
No answer came.
None.

4.

Other Factors

I don't know myself. This is what I am most often accused of. While I have seen the fields in my mind that I paint images of.

While I have toured studios where my dreams are woven with photos from various times of the day with differing tones because of the time or season of the year.
While I have taken walks among the ducks and the violently arranged wildflowers:

I'd always pick the ripest and readiest fruit from the bushes and trees. Constantly, quietly in Thanksgiving prayer even though you're not there.

In isolation I'd paint the phrase 'the mist crawls from the canal', using the act itself as an excuse to be alone. I'd sleep when tired. Eat when hungry. Paint my scene as deep, wide and tall as possible while listing all of the reasons why you're not with me.

Why I'm not enough. Why I'm nothing.

The painting I'm staring at might make me into something. The eating. The sleeping. The being tired. The brush-strokes. The cooking. The dreaming. The listing of 'things' (that are not things because they are more important than what 'thing' suggests) that mean you are a 3-message friend. Beyond that I will try and find myself amongst the *jouska* (imagined conversations) and the painting and the walking and the talking and 'other factors' where the more I become something I recognise as myself, the more likely I will finally write something 'worthwhile' as you suggested. That is what this is.

———

It was very dark. I could not sleep. The 11 on the wall meant it was closer to midnight than lunchtime. I would not see the sun for hours. It was December. I remember that part. The officer that drove me from the interview asked me what I had planned for Christmas. I reminded him that I was living in a place that gave me pills and checked on me in the middle of the night. Every night. To see if I was alive. Awake. There or actually *all there.* As in I knew where I was.

I'd been arrested but they hadn't used cuffs. I needed to explain money that had gone missing. Well, money someone had wired me as a deposit for some work. Work I'd never completed.

I'd disappeared. They thought I'd absconded and taken their money. So I was accused. And I was arrested. I was interviewed. I was ridiculed. I was humiliated. Then I was let go.

Taken back to the place where all I needed was books and clean pyjamas. Where I was being assessed. Where I was being asked to explain why I thought I didn't exist.

The interview room was cold and taupe. The table was stained and while I was offered tea, I was introduced to my advocate. A professional who was meant to ensure my wellbeing and safety during the interview. Later she sat quietly while the officer laughed after I answered his question: 'What's wrong with you?'

'I don't know who I am, and a wolf follows me everywhere I go so I'm scared.'

He was my age and thinner and shorter and he spoke with very little focus. He seemed to want to confuse me by showing me text messages and photos. His only plan was to get me to submit. I could not do that. He did not understand that he could not hurt me. I was incapable of feeling pain anymore.

He told me my name and then that there was no wolf. Even as I felt the hot breath against my neck and the saliva dripped onto my leg from pristine fangs. He followed his claim that there was no animal in the room with them by asking me 'Is there?'

As though I was a child being reminded that an adult version of the truth is always the truth.

My father used to look at me as though he was about to hurt me when he asked 'Isn't there?' My advocate just watched.

I realised he'd never known my brand of fear. A father who tried to kill me with alcohol and a car (on another occasion). His beatings were just warnings.

A mother who tried to kill me. With a Bible. With a campaign where she didn't speak to me at all. I'd respond by not speaking to her for twice as long. As soon as I could, I'd lied about my age and got as far away from them as possible.

As a result, it took a wolf that followed me everywhere to make me fearful enough to forget what I was and why I was where I was or who I was meant to be. The wolf was someone's deity. It became my north star. If it was 'there', I knew I wasn't anywhere at all. That I was lost. It reminded me – at these moments – that no one was looking for me.

When I was arrested, it was the first time anyone had looked for me. They wanted to know where their money was. I returned it the following week. No delay in that process. It was a simple misunderstanding.

Actually, I had no idea what they were talking about and all I know is that I was asked to pay £900 to avoid going to jail and I paid it. Frankly it felt like standard operating procedure for a place that made it clear that there was nothing wrong with me. Yet I was not allowed to leave.

Months later, as I lay in post-op recovery, my abusive accuser told me she knew the police officer. I didn't tell her that she'd gotten the name wrong. That what she'd described was false. That I was simply a toy for people to play with. A year later she said when it came to me, she'd 'loved and lost'. I realised at that moment that 'hated and found' were words I could not relate to either. I was equally lost and found.

I don't know me.

5.

A dear friend once challenged me with 3 questions:
Where do I live?
Who do I love?
What do I do?

Since their initial approach, I have answered the questions for myself many times. Every morning actually. Every. Morning. I once answered: 'Zug. No one. And change everything'. 4 years later, I can only answer 1 of those questions.
 For a short time 2 years ago, I could answer all 3. Yet, they were not the right 3.

I can always tell you what I want to do. I can't always answer 1 and 2. Sometimes I can lie but out of respect for my friend and the pointlessness of mornings I don't, and I simply allow 3 words out to puzzle myself: 'I don't know.'

Their questions are very straightforward. Practical like this friend, and without overthinking it, I can answer them on the sunny days. On the dark days when I succumb to F. Scott Fitzgerald's 3 a.m.[26] I can't answer at all or with anything but a lie. These are the times when I can only make lists of possibilities or outright lie, thus proving in so many ways that there isn't a single version of me someone can latch onto.

Or is there? I don't know. I gravitate toward there being more than 1 me.

While that may be true in a casual sense for everyone, I'm referring to a more complex model beyond the clichés of the 'work' me and the 'Saturday night' me. I am writing about the 'physical' me. The 'betrayed' me. The 'nimrod' me.

6.

The physical me

I stepped out into the warm air almost thick and accompanied by clouds pregnant with mid-summer rain. I did not stretch. I didn't take a deep breath. I don't think I did anything but start: 1 foot in front of the other toward an empty field where a man stood by a memorial marking a tragedy at a small school. He had flowers in his hand and stood grinding his teeth. I didn't go any closer. I was reminded of the Italian tourists at Auschwitz.

I literally jogged on. For 11 miles. I passed rolling fields and houses that got bigger and further and further apart. I galloped towards and through Glen Eagles (about to host the Ryder Cup). As night fell, I was overjoyed by the

---

[26] In a real dark night of the soul it is always three o'clock in the morning, day after day.' F. Scott Fitzgerald

‒‒‒‒

moon. By the time I stopped to rest, I'd run 45 miles in 9 hours. A personal best. For distance (the point) as opposed to speed, (which is relative because of age).

I could not sleep. I sat barefoot by the loch. Next to where the water rocked itself gently against a moored rowboat. It was 3am.

Since that morning, I have run faster and further and slower and shorter yet always with a sense that it has meaning to me and only me. I've run 210 miles in 7 days. I ran 235 in 7 the following year. I'm still hoping to get to 300. I've finally learned that it doesn't matter about the time, so I'm getting ready now.

That morning by the loch, though. With the wild future ahead of me, I didn't know how insignificant speed was and how important time is. Instead, I thought about what would help me sleep.

I came across something new. I only run for 1 reason. To feel empty. For however long I can escape into *something I can feel moving me like music across the bars. I'm swept up by the crescendo, which rises above everything until I am dropped into the valley where I sink to the lowest point, the nadir. Where I am my national insurance number and a body in a bed. Possibly clogging up the works. Where if my mind wasn't my enemy, then this bed I'm lying in with fresh scars would be free and then a surgical bed could be opened up to someone waiting anxiously at home. The fugue takes hold of me, abruptly pulling me from 1 movement to another.*

I remember apologising to the doctors because if I didn't exist then I wouldn't be such a nuisance. Apologies met with a silence that reminded me of my circumstances.

7.

The medicine makes it hurt

A young nurse had her hand on my chest as she poured a liquid drug into my mouth. It was chalky against my lips and then sweet at the back of my throat. Apparently the pain had woken me up and she'd found me in a ball on the floor. My IVs ripped out. I didn't know where I was.

A young man told me that the consensus was that I'd had a panic attack. That actually it would turn out to be something obvious and remedied with surgery. Pain, apparently, is alive in the mind and then lies dormant in the body, like giants in the hills before mythic wars.

Another man told me everything would be okay and that he'd be operating on me.

A woman told me the tumour was 7.5 millimetres in diameter.

2 young men kneeled at my bedside and told me that it was called cancer.

I received flowers from a young woman I'd thought had died.

Someone suggested I was okay because I was lucid. I could write. I could also sleep. What I couldn't do was stop the wolf from sitting on my chest.

It all felt as though something was ending. It all felt as though something was starting. Nothing felt warm.

The most clarifying detail? They sent a woman to ask me questions every day. Why didn't I have any more family?

——

Why had I simply just appeared bleeding internally? Where was I from?

They wanted to know who I was. My father was white and English. So my mother was clearly not at least 1 of those things, and possibly not either. My birth certificate and NI number notwithstanding, the woman who refused to give her name asked me who I was.

She meant what I was. I am not white. I am not Black. I am not Asian but she wasn't sure if Egyptian was African or Asian. She would have to check.

I explained that my Jamaican mother had Catalan ancestry and before that Egyptian. She reminded me of my ex-wife explaining to her Iranian aunts that my North African heritage meant I wasn't Black as they nodded in approving unison.

I momentarily became Jamaican until I produced a UK passport and reminded her of my birth certificate.

Her tone 1 day reminded me of Anthony DeMilio who, in 1978 asked me if I preferred 'Zebra' or 'Oreo' when I needed to explain that I wasn't Black even though my mom was.

She needed to define me. For her clipboard. For her statistics. She spoke to no one else. Every day she simply reminded me that what I was, was more important than who I was.

Or where I was going.

8.

After that I travelled somewhere outside of London alone. I checked into a hotel. I went to the hospital. I returned to the hotel. Apparently, what they'd removed was the source of all of my pain.

I recovered. I ate. I slept. I trained. I worked. I took the pills my GP had prescribed for the post-operative pain. The dullness that ended with sharp blows to my sternum.

I woke up alone. I woke up with sounds of soft tears hitting the marble floors with heating underneath. I fell asleep with the sound of something thumping in the distance. I walked around a city hoping that I wouldn't get lost again.

Then I woke up in a surgical bed. A young woman asked me if I was able to see a doctor. The pills, the ones my GP insisted would help, had given me blackouts. Banned in the US under a different name and originally meant to treat seizures of varying degrees, their ability to relieve pain was incidental.

I had lost a lot of blood.

After weeks of speculation, I was released to a community system that simply checked to see if I was alive and engaged with reality. The pain returned as soon as they stamped me as 'okay'.

The pain in my chest was sharper than ever. The shortness of breath had become panting. I never knew what day it was. I never knew what time it was. I started bleeding internally. I remember thinking there is no way anyone will think I'm not having a genuine event of some kind.

I'd been turned away after panic attacks for 2 years at this point. I'd been asked to take an HIV test. I didn't understand what was happening to me because the prevailing theory was that despite its very real consequences, I was inventing it. Nothing was conclusive until the blood was flowing. They'd need to remove half of my stomach. That's what they were all meeting about. That's why I couldn't be discharged. I had a growth that meant I was doomed.

I knew what had happened. There are these ghouls. They'd swallow all of the energy or life force a person had. They were *Ubir*. Or Incubus. This is where the vampire myths emerged from.

I'd become something like them. Eating other people's grief and pain. Relieving them of their burdens. I'd sucked the pain from their bones as I would have marrow from their souls. Or is that the other way around? I'd swallowed the wolf that chased me everywhere.

What they wanted to remove was from my mind and planted to grow like a tree in my body. The roots tearing through my muscles and sinews relentlessly. There was nothing they could do. Finally, I was doomed. I accepted everything I could by writing a list. I felt relief.

The Middle

'I accept that I chose not to communicate and you do not know why. I know this is a tautology. Something inescapable.'

'I accept that my penchant for allegories, metaphors and puzzles means you might not have known the real me.'

'I accept that it is your prerogative as to whether you communicate with me.'

'I accept that I am actively choosing not to communicate with you.'

'I accept there is nothing to forgive because the way I feel means there's no room for needing acknowledgement from you.'

'I accept that I am not expressing any of this to you.'

I remained undiagnosed. I was, at last, free from the wolf though. It had wandered into the forest and never returned. I had not been chained to it. He had been tethered to me. When I stopped wanting to know what was wrong with me and simply accepted what I could about the world I'd created for myself? That's when I felt free enough. When I felt I was not about to be devoured.

CHAPTER CONTRIBUTORS

DOLLY SEN
Dolly Sen is a disabled, working-class queer who has a brain of ill-repute that wants to disrupt systems that hurt people, not through trojan horse viruses but with my little ponies on acid with a little sadness in their hearts. Because of this she is a writer, artist, performer and filmmaker. Ten of her books have been published, she has written several chapters for academic publications, penned work for both theatre and film, and their subversive blogs around art, disability and humour for Disability Arts Online have a huge international following. She did some work in mental health archives and found only a small percentage was of the survivor voice so that's why she started this project. Dolly currently resides in Norwich. She/They.
www.dollysen.com

CONNE ARTIST (pen name)
Conne is a multi-disciplinary artist and raconteuse who takes inspiration from their own lived experience which is oh so very common to other marginalised and racialised folk around the planet yet exotic to the ruling classes. Conne artist enjoys centring suppressed marginalised voices thus liberating the healing and creative energy they encapsulate. These quashed narratives contain urgent messages and real solutions to our world's most pressing problems, namely: inequalities, climate justice and the way we treat the most vulnerable amongst us. Conne Artist mines these diamonds and shines a light on the beauty that she encounters there.

DAVE SOHANPAL
I can say I am an artistic person that was labelled trouble maker in class from a very young age, which later is known to be that I was dyslexic. Been through some

horrific traumatic experiences both in his home country and here in the UK. Thru is community and support who has helped him go thru all the tribulations and adversity.

DELE OLADEJI

is a British born Poet/Writer based in the Borough of Tower Hamlets, London. His collection of poems have been published by erbacce-press based in Liverpool, by the charity MIND and on the WEA website. His short poems have also featured in the Big Issue Magazine. He has written reflective pieces for ELFT (East London Foundation Trust), the People Speak and the Metro Newspaper. In 2019 he completed a MA in Creative Writing at the University of Westminster in London. He has since published more poetry published by erbacce-press. His last publication, 'The Sanatorium Voices' was used by Tower Hamlets Recovery College Book Club for students/service users.

Dele has worked as an actor; a career that started in Nigeria. He has done stage, television and radio works. Dele is a Befriender with ELFT. He is very passionate about Mental Health, and how creative writing can impact change, recovery and stability. He contributes regularly on various projects: the BAME focus Group, People Participation and Transformation team, ARIADNE Project, and the PPIE Project. Dele's short play, 'Reign Of Equal Rights' is currently streaming at Cardboard Citizens Theatre Company's' website. Dele currently works for the National Theatre in London.

CASSANDRA LOVELOCK

Cassandra (Cassie) Lovelock is a Black mixed race wheelchair user based in London. They are a writer, editor, speaker, and scholar activist who works and makes content across fields including mental health and neurodiversity, unpaid care, critical disability studies, and race studies.

She has bounced around various universities including King's College London, public sector bodies including NHS England, and third sector organisations challenging traditional knowledge hierarchies and centring and platforming lived experience stories from communities who are traditionally ignored by those in power. She/They @ soapsub across the internet.

A.PEONY (pen name)

I was drawn to sharing my experience in this book, as too often are our voices and experiences ignored or erased. Expressing one of the many harmful experiences at the hands of the system is incredibly important to me. To cast a light onto what really goes on within the system, so that the wider world is aware of what goes on and the injustice and discrimination we experience.

MIKLOTH BOND

My name is Mikloth Bond, I am a man in my 70s, of Caribbean decent, but have lived in the UK from the age of 7. Leaving Guyana, my birth country to come to England, proved very traumatic, and as a consequence I had no attachment to my parents when I arrived. Although I was unaware of it, I have experience mental health issues ever since then, only receiving a diagnosis in my late twenties. And after spending over 40 years in and out of mental health institutions, I finally got a grip on my mental health situation and am now finding my Voice, as someone who has lived most of their lives within the system.

The piece that I wish to submit is a document I prepared for a CMHT review I attended in April 2018. The document shows the desperate attempt of a man who has become aware that the system in which he had put his trust in for most of his life, was failing him, and that he needed to take control, by pleading for the CMHT to take another look at his diagnosis, and help him to be able to participate in his own rehabilitation. Only to be told after, his allotted half an hour, that CMHT don't do rehabilitation.

ANNA SMITH
I see myself as a survivor of psychiatric services. My journey has been difficult and even more of a struggle to find a direction for my life. I don't think I am someone who ever knew what they wanted to do with their life. I always enjoyed art at school, so I think I made that my starting point, hoping that I would eventually find my way. Now, I am applying to do an MA.

I am grateful for the fact that I have carried on having an interest in creativity during these confusing and painful years. It has helped me more than I ever realised.

JACQ A
is a Black, bisexual, nonbinary, fat, disabled writer and activist. Jacq has worked with several community groups including charities that support victims of crime, people who are HIV+ and homeless people. Jacq was the co-founder of Bisexuals of Colour, a social and support group that ran for 11 years, and produced the Bi's of Colour report - the only one of its kind in the world. Jacq is @SoOverTheRainbow on Instagram. Jacq's YouTube channel, Team Me, Team Us focuses on mental health for Abuse Survivors.

MICHELLE BAHARIER
is best known for founding CoolTan Arts, an Arts and mental health charity, famous for its Largactyl Shuffle Walks, Michelle's Midnight Walks took the audience on a vivacious live performance of myth and fact.

A graduate from the Slade School of Fine Art, Exeter College of Art & Design, an exchange student at Hochschule für Bildende, Künste Städelschule, Frankfurt am Main, Germany. She is available as a curator, workshop facilitator and she takes on public and private commissions.

Website: **https://michellebaharier.co.uk/**

Instagram: **Michelle Baharier - multi-media artist** or just put @bahariermichelle

Twitter: **Michelle (@dyslxicRant)**

LinkedIn: **Michelle Baharier FRSA - Artist - Freelance**

PRISCILLA EYLES

(she/they) is passionate about raising awareness of the issues neurodivergent and Disabled people with multiply marginalised identities like them face. Alongside destigmatising and demystifying topics like marginalised vulnerability to cult abuse and career trauma (particularly interested in highlighting abuses of so-called 'humanitarian' sectors like the charity sector), intergenerational/attachment trauma and intersectionality; as a racialised, neurodivergent queer person and cult survivor, and as advocate, speaker, JEDI (Justice, Equity, Diversity & Inclusion) trainer, writer and disability job coach.

They are currently trustee for Camden Disability Action and as well as the advocacy JEDI stuff, life model, babysit cats, do improv, tai chi, play the cello, sing and dance a lot (obsessed with ballet and tap dance).

Twitter: @PriscillaEyles, Insta: @CulturalLiasons

LinkedIn: linkedin.com/in/priscillaeyles   Music: dandylionuk.bandcamp.com/album/be-perfect   Email: **priscillaeyles@gmail.com**

C. BILN

I'm a person of south Asian descent and I don't get to read or hear much about people who have had similar experiences – though I am fully aware they exist in the world.

Mental health is something I really care about. Because of what I do and the sector in which I work, you can see its impact from the tiny kids I teach to their parents and grandparents. For me, it's really important to make more people aware of it because good mental health is the cornerstone of a really positive and happy life.

Resources are not always easily available or culturally specific to people's needs, and when you're at a really low point in your mental health, you do not want to do all the additional work that is required to get any support. Hopefully what this does is illustrate how hard getting support actually is – it should not be on the shoulders of those who are struggling.

I know when I don't have bandwidth, all of this unnecessary admin is even more of a burden; organising doctors' appointments, filling out paper work, and spelling out my name time and time again.

Stories like these are important, and while I am glad to have contributed mine, I am curious to learn about other peoples' experiences. I know I will be grateful for the sense of kinship.

S. KRAFTOWITZ

I'm Saskia Kraftowitz (they/he/she). Performing artist, agitator and researcher // Jewish Queer. I make stage sensations, street interventions, gallery interruptions and written publications. My practice spans genres, incorporating clowning, activism, dance, writing and nature conservation.

I take a solidarity approach working with gender expansive and multi-faith inclusion, acknowledging the social disability model and cultivating climate and ecologically sensitive creativity.

NINA OSEI WILSON

Ninette is a Peer Support Worker and Founder of Black Thoughts - an online support group for women of colour. Having spent over 3 years in the mental health field and over a decade pursuing a career in the creative industries, her ultimate aim is to obtain a MA in Art Psychotherapy to bridge this gap.

DAVID MARTIN ALEXANDER JOHNSTONE

prefers to be called Martin by the people he cares most about. Anyone who calls him David is probably from the United States where he has spent half his life. It is okay though. At this point they are lifelong friends.

In fact, by the age of 10 he had lived in 3 countries with various members of a family scattered across the globe. He has lived in over 50 houses and as a result has never really understood the concept of home. He is the son of a nurse and a teacher but always wanted to be a writer. He was 4 when he asked for a library card. The librarian at Glen Oaks Library said "If he can sign his name then he can have a library card". Martin practiced his signature for a week. It took until he was 6 to discover Edgar Allen Poe. At 18, while matriculating high school in Florida he was asked to explain what he wanted to do.
"See the world".
His explorer's spirit was already restless in his heart. When asked to explain why he said "So I have something to write about".

Mission accomplished. 32 countries later, for both work and pleasure, he has already self-published both fiction and non-fiction, won an award for his flash fiction and written a Country album that he performs at open mics and on social media. If you ask him what motivates him to be so eclectic. He will say "So that I will be remembered"

THE CUCKOO TEAM

PROJECT LEAD - DOLLY SEN

Dolly Sen is a disabled, working-class queer who has a brain of ill-repute that wants to disrupt systems that hurt people, not through trojan horse viruses but with my little ponies on acid with a little sadness in their hearts. Because of this she is a writer, artist, performer and filmmaker. Ten of her books have been published, she has written several chapters for academic publications, penned work for both theatre and film, and their subversive blogs around art, disability and humour for Disability Arts Online have a huge international following. She did some work in mental health archives and found only a small percentage was of the survivor voice so that's why she started this project.

Dolly currently resides in Norwich. She/They.
www.dollysen.com

EDITOR - DEBRA SHULKES (1975-2022)
Debra Shulkes was an editor and activist who struggled a bit with bios. She was a trauma survivor and a psych survivor: she can only write this because she's had the benefit of hearing and reading others' survival stories. Those stories filled her with words where there had been a hard silence.

Debra had been very lucky to have the chance to work on publications for the European Network of Users and Survivors of Psychiatry and the World Network of Users and Survivors of Psychiatry.
 She had been trained in international human rights frameworks by psych survivors and disabled people. She loved supporting people to take back their experiences and stories from those who have framed and silenced

them. She was part of (Re)-Imagining Mental Health Care, a Herstory memoir writing workshop for Mad-identified people.

EDITOR – CASSANDRA LOVELOCK

Cassandra (Cassie) Lovelock is a Black mixed race wheelchair user based in London. They are a writer, editor, speaker, and scholar activist who works and makes content across fields including mental health and neurodiversity, unpaid care, critical disability studies, and race studies. She has bounced around various universities including King's College London, public sector bodies including NHS England, and third sector organisations challenging traditional knowledge hierarchies and centring and platforming lived experience stories from communities who are traditionally ignored by those in power. She/They @ soapsub across the internet.

PRODUCER – CAROLINE CARDUS

Caroline Cardus is a visual artist and creative producer for disabled artists. She believes it is crucial for disability experiences to be part of mainstream arts culture, not just exist in a discrete, box ticking corner of life. In her art practice, Caroline makes work about the world disabled people live in. Through her work as a producer, she ensures disabled artists have a practical and creative ally to make bigger projects happen.

Caroline likes to work with Dolly because they both share a healthy belief in the power of the absurd – using subversion, mischief, and rage to reset false narratives of limits and disability, shame, and madness.

Thanks and Acknowledgments

DOLLY SEN: Firstly, the biggest thank you to my wonderful team: Debra Shulkes, Cassandra Lovelock and

Caroline Cardus for their big hearts and big brains. Debra, your death broke our hearts, but I still wouldn't have changed a thing, because this was what you wanted to do, and so many of the writers felt your love, care, and mighty mind.

Gratitude to the people behind the scenes, like my partner Alison Rose; James Peto, Melanie Grant, Solomon Szekir-Papasavva, and David Cahill Roots of Wellcome Collection; Jo Verrent, Ellie Liddell-Crewe, and Cat Sheridan of Unlimited; and every Lambeth librarian and library that saved my soul as a broken and mad teenager by showing me books can save your soul.

Thank you to the non-humans of the project, especially Scamp the dog and Barry the Llama.

Thanks to Anna Sexton who inspired my interest in archives, and much appreciation to Robert Dellar, who kick started my journey as a proud mad activist.

Thanks to the reviewers and foreword writers who gave their time, and our indexer, Kate.

Big love to all the authors of the books for sharing truth and life, and denying the bullshit told about our lives. I hope you all see the beauty of yourselves.

CAROLINE CARDUS: Thank you first and foremost to all the writers, who bravely shared some of their most painful experiences with us so generously so this book could be written.

Thank you to my partner Simeon Every, and my Mum, Barbara Cardus, who gave comfort, counsel, and support through some very tough times, and to my cats Halo and Bella (collectively known as The Orange Anarchy Society) who freely gave snuggles and purrs any time they were needed.

Ever grateful thanks to our editor Cassie Lovelock, for being a rock - in fact, a diamond, joining our team as an editor and friend, bringing great wisdom, gentleness, and even more animal photos.

Thank you is not nearly enough of an accolade to our dear late editor, Debra Shulkes, who died in October 2022 after a short illness. Even after her unexpected diagnosis, Debra spent some of the time remaining to her in editing writer's manuscripts. I'll never forget your dedication and selflessness, Debra, and I'll never forget all the laughs we had in project meetings, just because you went on holiday and got Barry the llama alpaca (who went on to become our official project mascot) drunk on fermented apples.

Thank you to Debra's cousin Gail Sulkes, her friend Nicola Robinsonova, and Debra's many dear friends, who helped myself, Dolly, and Cassie visit Debra in Prague and in whose company, we mourned her death. You all showed us such solidarity, community, and friendship in the aftermath of D's death – something none of us will ever forget.

My incredulous thank yous and constant amazement to Dolly Sen for daring to propose this project, and having the fierce, loving heart to see it through no matter what.

It has taken everyone involved in the project all their strength of will to place something so incredibly rare and incredibly important – survivor voices, at the heart of mental health debate and practice.

Thank you lastly to the readers who see the value of this.

CASSANDRA LOVELOCK: Thanks to all our authors, to all those who invested the time in untangling their stories for us to share; it has been the privilege of my life to work with each and every one of you. You have all given me far more than I will ever be able to repay but I hope having your words memorialised in these books goes even a small way toward all the healing that is deserved.

To Dolly, Caroline, and our dearest Debra, I feel so lucky to have worked together and so happy I sent that random email asking if I could join the team. Dolly, you helped me find and use joy as a way of wading through life. Caroline, your constant support, softness and solid helping of disability wisdom has taught me so much. And Debra, dearest Debra, I miss you terribly but know that I did my best to do these books in our honour knowing they will never be as good as if we could have worked together on them till the end.

Never ending thanks to my partner Dante and my friends for listening to me talk endlessly about this process, supporting me as I have grown as an editor and very much as a person.

Lastly, as with everything I do, this is for you, Ciera. You were never alone in your madness though I know you felt it. I hope you can be comforted from all these voices screaming about the injustices. I will never stop screaming for you.

DEBRA SHULKES: She didn't give us a list of people to thank before she died, but we know she loved the authors of the books and working with them. She'd want to thank each and every one of them. She would have wanted to say thank you to the people she spent her last days with. She loved her dad. She loved so many people. She loved the animals in and around her life. Hopefully, Debra, this is a good enough thank you.

———

GLOSSARY

The definitions given are the ideals. We, the authors, fully understand and acknowledge how the majority of these definitions do not adequately explain the variation in experience of mental health conditions

UK mental health system-related terms

CAMHS: Child and Adolescent Mental Health Services; CAMHS treat people primarily ages 18 and under

CMHT: Community mental health teams; CMHT provide treatment for people living with severe mental illness outside of hospital settings

CRHT: Crisis, or crisis resolution and intensive home treatment teams provide immediate acute support for someone in a mental health crisis who has not been admitted to hospital

CTO: Community treatment order; a tool used by clinicians to allow a person who has been detained in hospital to leave hospital and receive similar treatment in the community

DWP: Department for Works and Pensions; currently in control of the vast number of state welfare benefits including Employment Support Allowance, a means-tested disability benefit, and PIP (see below)

Forensic Services: Forensic mental health services specialise in the assessment, treatment, and risk management of people living with mental illness who are currently undergoing legal or court proceedings or are actively engaged in the criminal justice system.

IAPT: Improving Access to Psychological Therapies; The IPAT programme exists to provide people living with common mental disorders such as depression, anxiety or grief an easy way to receive therapies such as counselling or cognitive behavioural therapy. IAPT has recently been rebranded to NHS Talking Therapies.

Inpatient: A person who lives in hospital while receiving treatment

ITU, PICU: Psychiatric Intensive-Care Unit (PICU) or Intensive Therapy Units (ITU); specific wards in mental health hospitals which provide intensive assessment and treatment to those experiencing severe mental illness

Mental Health Act (1983): The first big piece of legislation which details people's rights in regard to treatment and assessment in hospital due to mental ill health

NICE: National Institute for Health and Care Excellence; NICE is a non-departmental government body that writes and publishes guidance for health and social care services on areas such as health technology, clinical practice and appropriate treatment methods and health promotion

PIP: Personal Independence Payment; PIP is a welfare benefit in the UK primarily for disabled people or those with long term health conditions.

OTHER IMPORTANT TERMS FOR UNDERSTANDING THE BOOKS

Ableism: Discrimination in favor of able-bodied people

Disableism: Discrimination against disabled people

ADHD: Attention Deficit Hyperactivity Disorder; a common neurodevelopmental disorder defined by disorganisation and problems prioritising, problems focusing and with multi-tasking, impulsiveness, and excessive activity.

Asexuality: Asexuality is the lack of sexual attraction to others, or low or absent interest in or desire for sexual activity.

Ace/Aro Spectrum: The range of experiences within Asexuality or Aromanticism.

Attachment theory: a psychological, evolutionary theory which describes how young children need to develop a relationship with a primary caregiver for 'normal/' social and emotional development. It explains the ways in which people that lack that secure attachment struggle into adulthood.

Autism: A lifelong developmental disorder defined by social communication and interaction challenges, over or under sensitivity to sounds, light, taste or touch, anxiety and meltdowns or shut downs, and special interests.

Body dysmorphia/Body Dysmorphic Disorder: A mental illness where a person experiences significant ongoing anxiety in relation to their appearance.

"BPD" construct: The argument that Borderline Personality Disorder is a political tool that psychiatry weaponises against particularly women who present as 'challenging' or 'manipulative.' Often these women have experienced significant trauma and/or are neurodivergent, but these experiences are ignored.

Cisgender: a person whose gender identity does match the one they were assigned at birth

Colourism: prejudice or discrimination against individuals based on their skin tone; typically among people of the same ethnic or racialised group

Dyslexia: a specific neurobiological learning disability which presents as difficulties with accurate and/or fluent word recognition and by poor spelling and decoding abilities.

Equalities Act: The 2010 Equalities Act in the UK consolidated all previous anti-discrimination law. Its three major statutory instruments include: protecting discrimination in employment on grounds of religion or belief, sexual orientation and age - but includes gender, disability, pregnancy status, and race/ethnicity

Gender dysphoria: Intense discomfort and distress experienced by those whose gender identity differs from their sex assigned at birth

Intersectionality: the interconnected nature of social categorisations such as race, class, and gender. Intersectionality explains how an individual can experience multiple overlapping layers of oppression and discrimination based on their social categorisations.

Invisible disability: A disability, chronic illness, or long-term health condition that has no obvious external markers on the body, or the disabled person uses no adaptive equipment that is associated with disability such as wheelchair or walking stick

Intergenerational trauma: a concept which aims to explain how trauma can be 'transmitted' through generations - particularly in response to traumatic events

LGBTQIA+ phobia: A term used to encompass the fear or dislike of someone, based on prejudice or negative attitudes, beliefs or views about people who are or are perceived to be Lesbian Gay Bisexual Trans Queer Intersex Asexual + with the plus meaning other identities that come under the LGBTQIA+ acronym

Neurodiversity: An umbrella term that refers to the diagnosable diversity of the human brain and cognition - it includes conditions such as ADHD, Autism, Dyslexia, and Tourettes syndrome

Non-binary: a person who identifies as a gender outside of 'man' or 'woman'

Misogyny: an ingrained or very strong prejudice against women

Misogynoir: a term used to show how sexism and racism manifest in black women's lives to create intersecting forms of oppression

Monogamous : the practice of having a single partner

Pansexual : a person who is attracted to people of all genders

Polyamorous (poly) : the practice of having multiple partners, all of whom are aware of and consent to the other relationships

Racism: prejudice and/or discriminatory treatment by an individual, community, or institution against a someone on the basis of their membership of a particular racial or ethnic group that is a minority or marginalised.

Racialisation: The process of the social construction of race; societies ascribe racial identities/social practices onto a group which did not identify itself in such a manner. Racilsation tends to arise from the dominant group ascribing a racial identity to a minority group for the purpose of othering and social exclusion.

Somatiser/Somatisation: Someone who presents with physical symptoms but have no biomarker or organic markers for the symptoms. Within mental illness, being labelled a somatiser often sees physical symptoms brushed off as 'all in your head' leading to struggles accessing support for physical needs.

Transgender : a person whose gender identity does not match the one they were assigned at birth

Transmisogyny: the intersection of transphobia and misogyny as experienced by trans women and transfem presenting people.

Transphobia: Originally Prejudice or discrimination against someone who is transgender. Now the term transphobia is used inclusive of violence and hate crime against someone who is not cisgender

With thanks to Bel Pye and Cassie Lovelock

Index

ALSO AVAILABLE

www.cuckoosnestbooks.co.uk